Secrets of a Healer

VOL. IV
MAGIC OF MUSCLE TESTING

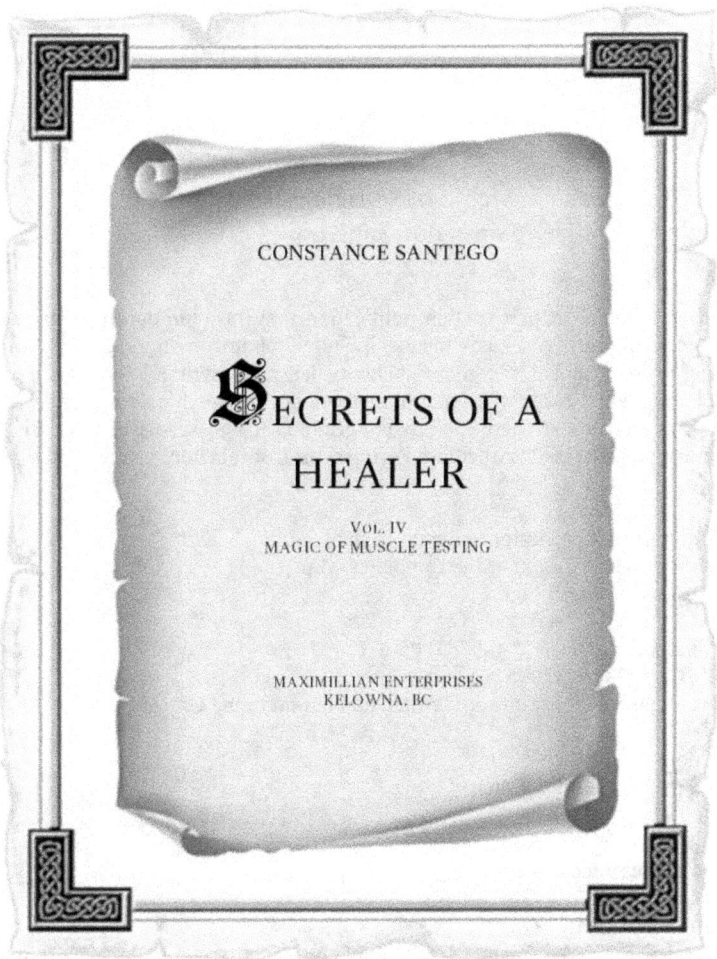

CONSTANCE SANTEGO

Secrets of a Healer

Vol. IV
MAGIC OF MUSCLE TESTING

MAXIMILLIAN ENTERPRISES
KELOWNA, BC

Secrets Of A Healer – Magic of Muscle Testing
Copyright © 2020 by Constance Santego.

All rights reserved. No part of this publication may be reproduced, distributed or transmitted in any form or by any means, including photocopying, recording, or other electronic or mechanical methods, without the prior written permission of the publisher, except in the case of brief quotations embodied in critical reviews and certain other noncommercial uses permitted by copyright law. For permission requests, write to the publisher, addressed "Attention: Permissions Coordinator," at the address below.

Copy Editor & Interior Design: Constance Santego
Book Layout: ©2017 BookDesignTemplates.com
Cover Design: Jennifer Louie

Trade Paperback ISBN: 978-0-9783005-3-1
Ebook ISBN 978-0-9783005-5-5
Created and published In Canada. Printed and bound in the United States of America

First Edition
Published by Maximillian Enterprises
Kelowna, BC
Canada
www.constancesantego.ca

Ordering Information:
Quantity sales. Special discounts are available on quantity purchases by corporations, associations, and others. For details, contact the "Special Sales Department" at the address above.

Dedication To The Holistic Women

Whom Brought Me Into
The Magical World Of Muscle Testing

My First Holistic Teacher, Diane Weibe
Touch For Health, Taught By Evelyn Mulders
Body Talk, Taught By Kristy Kenny
Aromatic Kinesiology, Taught By Robbi Zeck ND

Contents

Preface xi
Note to Reader xv
Learning Outcome xvii
PART ONE 19
BRIEF HISTORY 19
WHAT IS MUSCLE TESTING 21
    MERIDIANS 23
    MERIDIAN ABBREVIATIONS 26
    YIN & YANG 27
    TSUBO 29
    CHINESE BODY CLOCK 31
HOW TO MUSCLE TEST 35
    TESTING METHOD #1: Muscle Test the Arm 35
    TESTING METHOD #2: Body Pendulum: 37
    TESTING METHOD #3: Surrogate Person 39
    TESTING METHOD #4: Pulse Reading 40
    TESTING METHOD #5: Finger Lock: 44
    TESTING METHOD #6: Pendulum: 45
    TESTING METHOD #7: Paper: 49
THE SECRET IS... IN THE QUESTION 51
WHAT CAN YOU MUSCLE TEST FOR? 65
PART TWO 68
    HOW TO BALANCE YOUR BODY 68
    BONUS Exercise to Practice 69
    BALANCING METHOD #1 Quick Fix 70
    BALANCING METHOD #2 Meridian Walking 75
    BALANCING METHOD #3 Source Points 76

BALANCING METHOD #4 Strengthen / Weaken 77
BALANCING METHOD #5 Muscles Massage 92
BALANCING METHOD #6 Five Element Theory 96
HOW TO PERFORM A SESSION 113
OTHER QUESTIONS You Can Muscle Test: 117
EXTRA QUESTIONS: 121
    EMOTIONAL: 122
    MENTAL: 123
    PHYSICAL: 124
    SPIRITUAL: 142
BIBLIOGRAPHY 149
MESSAGE FROM THE AUTHOR 151

*Many times, brilliance is brought forward from the past;
our ancestors knew some of the best tricks and tips.*

—Constance Santego

Preface

The Miracle of Muscle Testing

Why Muscle Testing?

In 1993, I owned an industrial sewing and manufacturing company and all I did the first time my back went out was pick up a pencil from the floor.

I did go see a doctor, but my options were an operation or take pain killers for the rest of my life. At the time, my children were only three and four years old and the thought of becoming paralyzed stopped the operation. The long-term side effects stopped me from wanting to take the pills. I decided to give alternative medicine a try. Believe me, when you are lying on the floor in sheer pain and can't move you will try everything and anything to get better.

Massage Therapy called my condition an overuse injury. I had been doing the same heavy lifting while twisting motion for about fifteen years. This motion was continually putting too much tension on my lower back muscles, and they finally couldn't take the trauma anymore and allowed my vertebra to be pulled out of alignment.

I was able to keep mobile with two years of weekly visits to the Chiropractor. Unfortunately, this did not solve the problem it just made life bearable and I eventually had to face the truth that I needed to sell my business.

Within the next year, I started working in a holistic healing center and one of the first modalities I learned was Muscle Testing. I was in love with Muscle Testing! The techniques I learned changed my life; I now had a way to keep my muscles relaxed and my bones aligned without drugs or weekly Chiropractic sessions.

Dr. Goodheart, a 1960's Detroit Chiropractor, developed a technique for MD and Chiropractors called Applied Kinesiology. His protégé, Dr. John Thie, developed a lay person's system called Touch For Health (TFH). These modalities combine acupuncture theory with a variety of western discoveries that involved touch reflexes and Muscle Testing. Today there are many practitioners and courses that use a form of Muscle Testing for healing: Kinesiology, Touch for Health, Shiatsu, Reiki, Body Talk, Naturopathy or any other modality that uses chakras or meridians.

Traditional Chinese medicine the body is thought of as a whole being. It is understood that man is a structural, chemical, mental and spiritual being. If one system is out of balance, it is thought to affect the whole. The Chinese doctors improve the muscle by restoring the energy flow of these systems; this also gives relief to the organ which is sharing that system.

Meridians are invisible pathways for positive and negative energy (Qi, Chi, Prana) to flow through the body. There are twelve main meridians: Lung, Large Intestine, Stomach, Spleen, Heart, Small Intestine, Bladder, Kidney, Pericardium/Circulation /Sex, Sanjiao/Triple Warmer, Gall Bladder, and Liver. These pathways are different for each meridian; the meridian travels deep in the body and on the outside along the skin opposite paths on the left and right side of the body for each meridian.

Our skin's sensory system is so acute that we can notice the faintest breeze. Our brain is amazing; it can sense, retain, configure and respond in a split second. Our mind contains all the information about what is wrong in our bodies and how to fix it. We just need a way to comprehend an answer. A literal question is the most important part.

If you go to an alternative medicine practitioner, he/she may have used muscle testing to determine what and how to help you. There are a few different methods used. Some use a finger lock technique where the practitioner's thumbs and pointer fingers are linked together forming a figure eight. By trying to pull them apart, he/she will get a "yes" or "no" answer, "yes", being locked and "no" unlocking. Some practitioners use the client's arm as a lever, with "yes" being a solid or strong arm and "no", the arm is limp or let's goes.

If you are not responding, go to the washroom, drink water or zip-up three times (using your hand, pretend you are zipping upstart from the bottom of the torso and follow up to the lips 3x).

There are many different reasons why a person's meridian may be blocked. Physical, emotional, mental or spiritual injury, and the deeper or longer the person has had the issue, may determine the number of sessions needed.

In my own case, to take back control of my situation and to save me from an operation, I did these muscle testing techniques, and still due to this day just to stay healthy.

I use Muscle Testing for soooo many great and fascinating reasons…

Enjoy, Constance

Note to Reader

Muscle Testing is not to replace modern medicine; Your Doctor still plays a very important role in your health care. If I break my leg I definitely will want and need a Doctor and all the nurses and staff that work in the Hospitals to help me.

My perception of Eastern Medicine's belief is that we play a major role in taking care of our own health, not leaving it up to the doctors to fix us after the fact. Eastern Medicine is all about balancing the body, mind, and soul; reducing our stress level, creating a vital energy force, and watching what we put into our body and our mind.

Muscle Testing is a tool, a technique that permits our conscious mind to connect with our subconscious mind. If you develop your sensitivity to answering your questions with honesty and integrity you will be on a path of wellbeing for your Body, Mind & Soul.

Shift happens…Create magic!

Learning Outcome

When you have completed this book and studied the concepts and techniques, you will;

- Know the basics of Muscle Testing.
- Develop seven testing methods to get answers to not only your questions about your body but to receive answers for your mind & soul as well.
- Have many balancing methods that will help you achieve chi. . . balance. One of which is a quick pain relief technique.
- Basics of using the Five Element Theory.
- An amazing list of specific questions that you can muscle test for yourself to heal your physical, mental, emotional, and spiritual body.

PART ONE

BRIEF HISTORY

Applied Kinesiology

Muscle Response Applied Kinesiology originated in 1964 by Dr. George Goodheart (Chiropractor). He started with pressing on the Origin and Insertion of a muscle and progressing to testing a muscle's strength or weakness by moving the body parts in the direction of the muscle movement towards the origin; weak muscle - issue, strong muscle - no issue.

Later tested for diagnosing conditions- 1) the nervous system 2) the lymphatic system 3) the vascular (blood vessels) system 4) the cerebrospinal fluid 5) the meridian system…Holistic Practitioner – Chemical, Mental and Structural balance.

Trigger Point Therapy

Stemmed from Applied Kinesiology.
Cycle: Person has pain – Muscle tension – reduced circulation – muscle shortening – creating restricted movement. Trigger Point Therapy is based upon a Nodule/Knot point which can cause referred pain to another location (tight muscles, spasm or opposing muscles/opposite muscle). Relief of pain is created by a Chiropractor or a Massage Therapist finding a Nodule/Knot and push and rub it until it disappears.

Touch for Health

Using Applied Kinesiology with the understanding that Quoted from John Thie, DC, "Some muscles are related to a specific organ system because they share a lymph vessel or an acupuncture meridian."

John Thie, DC developed a forty-two-muscle balance modality, Touch for Health, using the Applied Kinesiology technique of moving the specific muscle towards its origin to test if it is weak or strong and then using one of the balancing techniques

Body Talk

The BodyTalk System was developed by Dr. John Veltheim in 1996 and combines aspects of modern physics, traditional Chinese medicine, East Indian philosophy, applied kinesiology, and Western medicine.

The BodyTalk System™ is a healing modality that allows the energy systems of the body to be synchronized so that the body can function as it is meant to. No diagnosis is given, nor medications prescribed. It is non-invasive, no contraindications to its use and is totally safe

WHAT IS MUSCLE TESTING

As many of you know this is one of the courses, I use to teach my students who were becoming holistic healers. I am very excited to be sharing with you one of the most amazing techniques used for personal and clinical healing.

As a Holistic Practitioner, we do not treat diseases or symptoms, only a medical doctor can do that. We balance stress of the body, mind, and soul; by using natural healing modalities and techniques such as Muscle Testing.

In the past, only Kinesiologist, Chiropractors, Physiotherapist, and Massage Therapists used the technique of testing an individual muscle to ascertain if that muscle needed balancing. If so, proceeding to balance that muscle by either relieving the stress and tension or by improving its strength.

Today, based on the belief that the subconscious mind knows all that is needed to heal the body. Muscle Testing is more commonly used by many Alternative, Integrated, and Natural Health Practitioners, to determine a yes/no answer to a very specific question relating to the client's Emotional, Mental, Spiritual or Physical wellbeing.

The wisdom of Western Muscle Testing combined with the Eastern genius knowledge of meridians and chakras is considered a paradigm shift in the healing world!

In this book, by using one of the seven taught Muscle Testing methods; you will learn how to determine which of the meridians/organs/muscles that need balancing AND/OR how to ask a specific question for the purpose of Homeostasis.

If you know how to perform massage, there is a portion at the end of the book which has charts of specific muscles that correlate with the body's organs and meridians.

Enjoy balancing your body!

P.S. Back in 1997, Muscle Testing was one of the very initial courses that I learned, and at first, I only memorized how to do the quick fix balancing technique to relieve pain. As simple as the three-minute technique is, people were astonished at how they felt after rubbing these specific points.

Constance

MERIDIANS

Meridians, acupressure vessels or channels are invisible pathways for positive and negative energy (Ki, Qi, Chi, Prana, Life force energy, etc.) to flow through the body; connecting the organs, skin, flesh, muscle, and bones.

There are fourteen meridians that run through your body and are mainly associated with the organs. These pathways are different on each meridian, the meridian flowing deep in the body and on the outside along the skin (but not at the same time).

There are two special meridains, Ren (aka central or conception vessel) and Du (aka governing vessel). Plus, the other twelve: Lung, Large Intestine, Stomach, Spleen, Heart, Small Intestine, Bladder, Kidney, Pericardium (aka circulation/sex), Sanjiao (aka triple warmer), Gall Bladder, and Liver.

You may have heard of Acupuncture. Oriental medicine has been using these meridian pathways for centuries. The Chinese consider the meridians to be the web of life. They believe that vital energy circulates through these channels, nourishing all systems of the body.

According to the ancient Chinese teachings, these "rivers of health" flow continuously through the body. It was believed that a person would become sick when his meridians were blocked.

There are many different reasons why a person's meridians may be blocked. Stress is a big reason. Meridians may also be blocked at one time and not at another.

- A person may have had a <u>physical</u> injury and the trauma is too much for his system to handle or is protecting him from further harm. For example, a broken arm may take months to heal and his meridians will correspond.
- A person may have had an <u>emotional</u> injury and the upset is too

much for the system to handle. For example, a memory may be blocked, or the person may have been driving and in his past, he had another vehicle almost hit him so it would take his system time to recoup.
- A person may have had a <u>mental</u> injury. For example, a teacher or an accountant might never have time to just "zone"; he is "on" at all times and this may lead to a nervous breakdown or other physical issues.
- A person may have had a <u>spiritual</u> injury. For example, a person may have a near-death or religious experience.

The deeper the issue, the more layers of the onion you may have to peel, which means this person may need many sessions to balance his meridians. Acupressure, Acupuncture, Kinesiology, Touch for Health, Shiatsu, Reiki or any other discipline that uses chakras is based on this same meridian system belief.

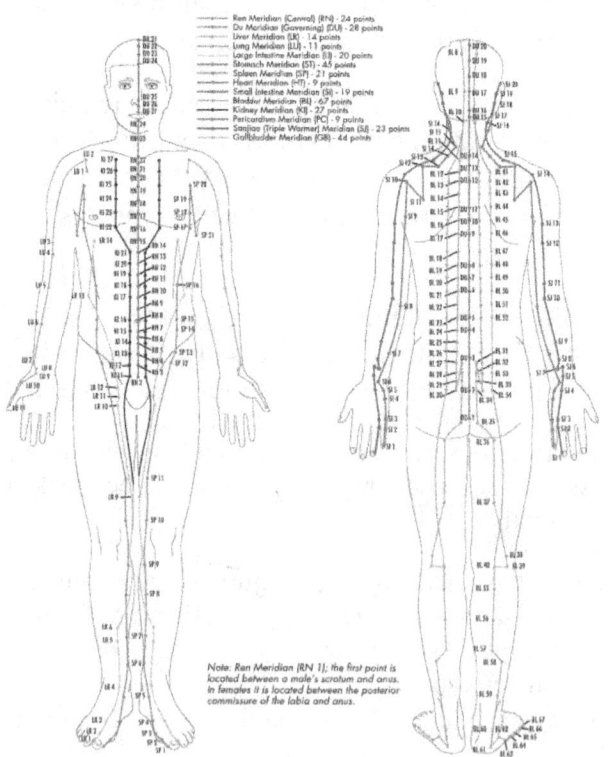

FIGURE 1: Anterior View of Meridians   FIGURE 2: Posterior View of Meridians

Note: Ren Meridian (RN 1); the first point is located between a male's scrotum and anus. In females it is located between the posterior commissure of the labia and anus.

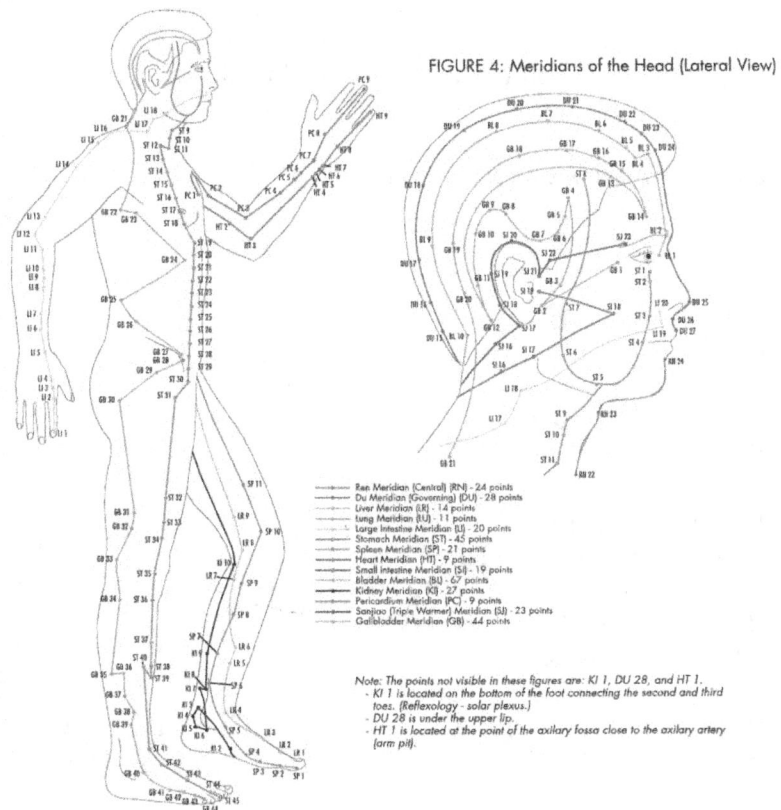

FIGURE 3: Lateral View of Meridians

FIGURE 4: Meridians of the Head (Lateral View)

Note: The points not visible in these figures are: KI 1, DU 28, and HT 1.
- KI 1 is located on the bottom of the foot connecting the second and third toes. (Reflexology - solar plexus.)
- DU 28 is under the upper lip.
- HT 1 is located at the point of the axillary fossa close to the axillary artery (arm pit).

MERIDIAN ABBREVIATIONS

Any Acupuncture Points Chart will display all the meridians and tsubo points on the body.

Permachart.com is an excellent chart to view

LU	Lung		
LI	Large Intestine		
ST	Stomach		
SP	Spleen		
HT/H	Heart		
SI	Small Intestine		
BL/B	Bladder		
KI/K	Kidney		
PC/P	Pericardium	or	C/S Circulation /Sex
SJ	Sanjiao	or	TW Triple Warmer
GB	Gall Bladder		
LR/LV	Liver		
RN	Ren Meridian	or	CV Conception Vessel / Central
DU	Du Meridian	or	GV Governing Vessel /Governing

YIN & YANG

Meridians are categorized into two groups;

Yin meridians

- Flow up the body
- Are located on the inside of the arms and legs, and on the front of the body.

Yang meridians

- Yang meridians flow down.
- Are located on the back, the sides of the body, the head, and the outside of the arms and legs (An easy way to remember, a man protects - Yang energy is male, protecting our back).

Yin Meridians	**Elements**	**Yang Meridians**
Heart	Fire	Small Intestine
Spleen	Earth	Stomach
Lung	Metal	Large Intestine
Kidney	Water	Bladder
Liver	Wood	Gall Bladder
Pericardium /C-X	Fire	Triple Warmer

The forces of Yin & Yang interact constantly in all forms of life. Traditional oriental health care is based on the universal yin-yang laws which govern all changes.

The Yang Meridians (or channels) flow DOWNWARD on the backs of the arms & legs.

The Yin Meridians (or channels) flow up the front, inner surfaces of the body.

Yin & Yang Associations - The opposite of any situation...

YIN	YANG
Earth	Heaven
Female	Male
Shakti	Shiva
Space	Time
Stillness	Activity
Night	Day
Darkness	Light
Cold	Heat
Contraction	Expansion
Interior	Exterior
Falling	Rising
Soft	Hard
Rounded	Angular
Curved	Straight

TSUBO

A Tsubo is a specific point along the meridian. The different meridians have a different number of points that you can balance.

Lung	11 points
Large Intestine	20 points
Stomach	45 points
Spleen	21 points
Heart	9 points
Small Intestine	19 points
Bladder	67 points
Kidney	27 points
Pericardium or Circulation /Sex	9 points
Sanjiao or Triple Warmer	23 points
Gall Bladder	44 points
Liver	14 points
Ren Meridian or Conception Vessel / Central	24 points

The Tsubo can be; balanced, indented or excess (puffy) when you touch it.

" If the Tsubo is not balanced you may need to work on each tsubo point individually by **Tonification & Sedation (KYO & JITSU) technique**. " The condition of energy (chi or ki) in the meridians is defined by *KYO and JITSU*.

KYO (pronounced KEYO) is the condition of depleted /deficient energy, which is more *hypo*.

" The technique used to normalize kyo points is called *tonification*.

" The hollow areas (indents) of kyo require patient holding. This takes more time because warmth must reach deep inside to nurture the area.

" To tonify a point, use clockwise rotations.

JITSU *is* the condition of excess energy, which is more *hyper*.

" The technique used to normalize jitsu points is called *sedation*.

" In sedation, the jitsu area is simply stimulated and the protrusion will normalize itself.

" To sedate a point, use counterclockwise rotations.

The following diagrams illustrate the conditions of KYO and JITSU

Balanced

Kyo

Jitsu

An easy way to remember:
Kyo / hollow/ o'clock (clock wise)

CHINESE BODY CLOCK

When a Meridian is working the hardest and when it is resting/not working hard at all.

Lung	3 – 5 AM
Large Intestine	5 – 7 AM
Stomach	7 – 9 AM
Spleen	9 – 11 AM
Heart	11 AM – 1 PM
Small Intestine	1 – 3 PM
Bladder	3 – 5 PM
Kidney	5 – 7 PM
Pericardium	7 – 9 PM
Triple Warmer	9 – 11 PM
Gall Bladder	11 PM – 1 AM
Liver	1 – 3 AM

High tide is when the meridian is at its peak when it is working.

Low tide is 12 hours difference when it is resting.

Example: A person awakens to go to the bathroom (Bowels) between 5-7 AM (Large Intestine) = high tide. This is the optimal time to treat & supplement the Large Intestine. This person may become fatigued between 5-7 PM (opposite time, Kidney) = low tide.

- It is advised to receive treatments & take supplements between 5 and 7 AM, as well as between 5 and 7 PM. If this timing is not convenient, help at any time of the day or night will be better than nothing.

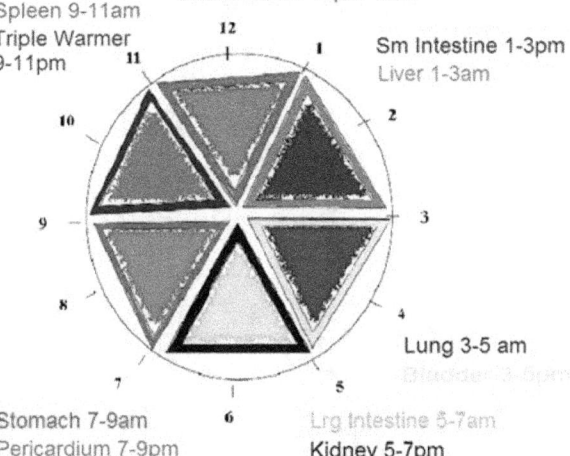

Chinese Body Clock — Followed by Acupressure/Acupuncture & Touch For Health

Heart 11am-1pm
Gall Bladder 11pm-1am
Spleen 9-11am
Triple Warmer 9-11pm
Sm Intestine 1-3pm
Liver 1-3am
Lung 3-5 am
Bladder 3-5pm
Stomach 7-9am
Pericardium 7-9pm
Lrg Intestine 5-7am
Kidney 5-7pm

Muscles

Liver	1-3am	Pectoralis major sternal, Rhomboids
Small Intestine	1-3pm	Quadriceps, Rectus abdominis,
Lung	3-5am	Coracobrachialis, Deltoid middle & posterior, Serratus anterior, Diaphragm
Bladder	3-5pm	Peroneus longus & brevis, Tibialis anterior & posterior, Erecta spinae group
Large Intestine	5-7am	Quadratis lumborum, Tensor fasciae latae, hamstrings
Kidney	5-7pm	Psoas, Illiacus *(Ileo-cecal valve)*, Trapezius upper *(Eyes & Ears)*
Stomach	7-9am	Pectoralis major clavicular, Sternocleidomastoid, Lavator scapula *(Sinuses)*, Brachioradialis
Pericardium/Cir/Sex	7-9pm	Adductors, Gluteus max & med, Piriformis
Spleen	9-11am	Latissimus Dorsi & Triceps brachii *(pancrease)*, Trapezius middle & lower, Opponens pollicis longus *(Thumb)*
Sanjiao/Triple Warmer	9-11pm	Adrenals = Sartorius, Garcilis, Gastrocnemius, Soleus
Heart	11am-1pm	Subscapularis
Gall Bladder	11pm-1am	Tensor fasciae latae, Quadratus lumborum *(spine)*, Popliteus, Anterior deltoid

Main Meridians

Ren / Central	8 pm	Supraspinatus *(Brain)*
Du / Governing	12 Noon	Teres major *(Spine)*

HOW TO MUSCLE TEST

TESTING METHOD #1:
Muscle Test the Arm

What to do: training another person's arm:

1) Hold the (left or right) arm straight out in front (or out to the side) and parallel to the floor.

2) To show/demonstrate a 'yes', ask him/her to "hold" (arm should be firm, not held with all his/her might but just a solid, straight arm which is parallel to the floor).

3) To show/demonstrate a 'no', ask him to let his arm drop to the side.

4) Show him <u>three</u> times what a yes and no is (you may have to literally hold his arm up for yes and move his arm down to the side for no. What you are doing is training/programming the mind.

5) Once the person understands the process, you test the arm; with your two fingers flat above the wrist bone, press with 2-pounds of pressure, with a 2-inch movement, for 2-seconds on the extended arm saying, " Arm firm means yes."

6) Now say, "Arm down is no.", while you press with your two fingers flat above the wrist bone, with 2 pounds of pressure, with a 2-inch movement, for 2 seconds on the extended arm. The arm should have dropped to the side.

If step 5 and 6 are not working, if he/she is **not responding** with the arm or body pendulum, have him drink water, or zip-up three times (Ren/Central Meridian: using his hand pretend he is zippering up, start from the bottom of the body and follow up to the bottom lip). He might also need to go to the washroom.

7) Do this action of yes/no and no/off about three times (3x) each. You are programming the person's mind to be able to answer you.

It may take you quite a few times to learn the pressure and to notice the arm being strong, not let go for a 'yes' and letting go, dropping to the side for a 'no'. The thinking of some people gets in the way so much that you may have to train them a few times or teach them body pendulum.

Apply firm pressure gradually and then release it gradually. The muscle will either be strong, or lock into place in the first few minutes of the test, or it will give way completely. Learn to feel the difference between a muscle that locks or a muscle that shakes and is giving way. A muscle that gives way is often described as feeling mushy. If a muscle hurts during the test, stop immediately, assume it is weak, and work to strengthen it.

TESTING METHOD #2:
Body Pendulum:

1) Have the person stand upright.

2) Have the person lean forward from the ankles saying, "Forward is a 'yes', without falling" (the person needs to remain stiff, like a board).

3) Have the person lean backward from the ankles saying, "Backward is a 'no', without falling."

4) Have the person repeat this movement back and forward three times to program the mind.

5) Have the person practice:

a) Have him say, "My (meaning the person's name) name is _____." If he goes forward, that is correct.

b) Then practice a fake name; if he goes backward, that is correct.

c) Do a few silly, obvious questions to train him. (e.g. "My shirt color is _____.)

d) Use vitamins; have the person hold the vitamins (still in the container) and ask, "Do I need to take any today?"

If the answer is *yes*, then how many? For how many days? Add anything else you can think of.

6) Have the person then answer any other questions needed.

Remember the mind is <u>very literal</u>; it will only answer literally what you asked.

If the body sways sideways,
ask a different or more detailed question;
if it stays still/does not move, it does not know an answer.

Vitamins are great to use while learning this because the vibratory rate is so high.

" Now ask this question while holding the vitamins to your stomach, "Is this vitamin(s) what my body needs to have today?" Make sure your knees are relaxed and are locked neither too tightly nor loosely, just comfortably. Now allow your body to move it will either go forward or backward for the 'yes' or 'no' answer. If your body goes side to side, it means you need to ask a more specific or a better question. Try this with 5 – 10 different kinds of vitamins. When you feel confident and you can tell the difference between 'yes' and 'no', try candy or your name (if you answer incorrectly to your name, make sure you say, "in this lifetime"), or ask any other very specific single answer question you want to be answered.

This tool can only be used with a 'yes' or 'no' answer.

Make sure you are very specific, after a dream I had I asked if I should move the school and it said 'no' but then I asked should I move all the contents in the school and it said 'yes'. The answers are always extremely literal. The building/school (bricks and wood) should not move.

When asking a personal question, make sure to ask for an honest and unbiased answer. It does not always work for your own questions. *Your conscious mind knows what answer you really want.*

TESTING METHOD #3:
Surrogate Person

If the other is not able to have you muscle test them, even after trying the first two techniques, have a second person act as a surrogate. Have him hold on to the original person, and then you now muscle test the second person *(surrogate person)* as if he was the original person. The surrogate person would have the intent of just being a filter for the original person. We are not testing the surrogate person's issues, only the original person's issues.

When you are muscle testing with a surrogate person, have the intent (think) of the original person only. All of the rest of the muscle testing technique information is the same.

TESTING METHOD #4: Pulse Reading

The Pulse In Comparison To The Five Elements

The nourishing cycle and the controlling cycle relationships can be felt in the pulses *(you will read shortly about this in more detail)*. On the right hand, we have the positions of the organs relating to the Fire, Earth and Metal elements, and on the left, we have Water, Wood, and Fire.

PULSE: Yang / Yin   Yin / Yang

Pulse Qualities

Speed: **Slow** (less than 4 beats per respiration)

Fast (more than 5 beats per respiration)

Strength: **Empty** (weak and soft)

Full (strong and pounding)

Shape: Is the pulse **slippery, choppy, wiry, tight and soggy**?

Rhythm: Is the pulse **hesitant, intermittent, knotted, relaxed and rapid** (> 90 beats per minute), **racing** (> 120 beats per minute), **skipping** (rapid and irregularly irregular)?

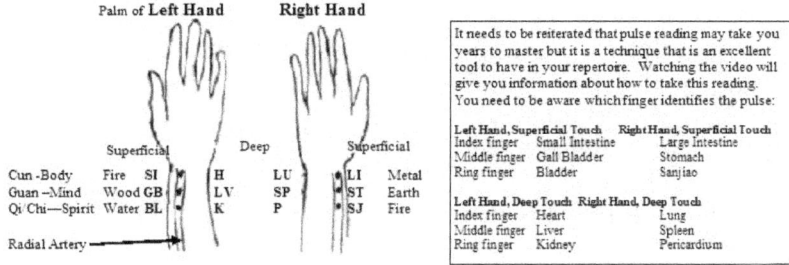

Pulse Reading

The best time to pulse test is early morning.

Have the person rest for five minutes after he comes in before reading the pulse.

Pulse: You will feel for the heartbeat/pulse on the person's arm. Put your index, middle and ring finger on the person's arm, starting where the wrist bend and just under the thumb (radial artery).

Test For Superficial Pulses- lightly touch just on the surface of the person's skin. Feel for a pulse. Wait a few moments (up to one minute). Do you feel any pulse? If yes, identify which meridian/organ from the picture on the previous page. Mark the information on a piece of paper or the client chart (off/on) and proceed to step 3. I have an example of the charts I use in this book.

Test For Deep Pulses- push into the arm a little bit. *If you press <u>too</u> hard, there will be no pulse.*

Mark the information down, the same way as with the superficial reading.

Pulse positions are relative to the person's body size and your finger size. Individuals' fingers vary in size so you will have to change/adjust your finger position to fit on the person's wrist.

Note:

> -An athlete's - normal pulse is slower than the average person
>
> -Women- pulse faster than a man's
>
> -Children- pulse is faster than that of adults
>
> - If someone is fat/heavy - slow and deep
>
> - If someone is very slim- superficial and rapid

Shape: Different Types of Pulses
(to sense the differences it could take you years)

Weak pulse - difficult to detect. *Meaning*-weak constitution, chi or blocked Yang / Yin

Strong Pulse - good form and resiliency. *Meaning*– strong constitution, no major deviancies, bounce back well.

Soft pulse - spreads & moves with pressure, feels moist. *Meaning*– spleen & kidney may be weak.

Floating pulse (wavy) - felt easy at the surface. *Meaning*- usually beginning of the disease, e.g. cold/flu

Sinking pulse - deep palpitations. *Meaning*– a constriction of the interior organs, constipation.

Thin pulse - feels thin/thready. *Meaning*– deficiency in the Yin, thirst, dry skin, constipation.

Full pulse - really there. *Meaning*- excess condition, requires sedation.

Tense pulse - bowstring. *Meaning* – presents some force, liver tension and common with restrained anger.

Fast pulse - *Meaning*– heat syndrome =inflammation thriving; thin weak pulse that is fast relates to Yin deficiency

Slow pulse - *Meaning*– cold syndrome= strong stagnancy of circulation; pain, lethargy, chills

Slippery pulse - (normal between 6-8 weeks of pregnancy) – firm + round pearls under the fingers. *Meaning*– phlegm accumulation, stagnation of moisture, digestion disturbed, mentally disturbed, nerves damaged.

Congestion pulse - slippery quality, but sinking; may not feel 3 finger pulse, *Meaning*– abdominal disturbances, congestion of phlegm or blood or deviancy of Yin.

TESTING METHOD #5:
Finger Lock:

1) Have the person interlock their one hand's pointer finger and thumb inside of the other hand's pointer finger and thumb (fingers should create a figure eight).

2) Have the person lock fingers as they pull apart, saying, "lock is a yes", do three times (3x)

3) Have the person unlock fingers as they pull apart, saying, "unlock is a no", do three times (3x)

4) Have the person repeat this movement lock and unlock three times to program the mind.

TESTING METHOD #6:
Pendulum:

(From My Published 'Intuitive Life' Book)

A pendulum is defined as a weight hung from a fixed point so that it can swing freely, and specifically refers to a rod with a weight at the end that regulates the mechanism of a clock.

The pendulum is tuned to your personal vibration by allowing the string to slip loosely through the *thumb, middle and pointer fingers* until it appears to rotate. The pendulum's string should be no longer than the distance of you are holding the string in your fingers and your elbow resting on a table; the pendulum should not hit the table.

Answers Using A Pendulum

There are many different ways a person can find the answers for which he/she is searching. This section focuses on how to receive answers for yourself or others.

- First, you must ask a literal question. The mind and creator/spirit is extremely literal. If you ask, "Can I help this person?" or, "Can I cure this person?" You will find that these are two very different questions. The words you use in your question will be interpreted literally. Our everyday language contains a lot of slang which is intended to have the same meaning as formal English but frequently this is not the case.
- The time frame is very important also. If you ask, "Can I cure this person?" and the answer is "yes", did you ask "Today?" Try to be specific and to the point. This may take a lot of practice.

- Write down your questions, so when you receive an answer you can re-check if you were specific enough.

You can buy a pendulum or make your own. A necklace will work also.

- To make a pendulum you will need:
    - Thread (gold or silver color elastic heavy thread works very well) or chain
    - Hot glue and gun or solder gun
    - Beads (one large oblong bead, metal cover, three to five smaller beads)
    -
- Procedure:
    1. Cut the thread to approximately 10 inches.
    2. Attach one end of the thread to the larger bead.
    3. Place metal or plastic cover over the larger bead and through the thread.
    4. Glue together.
    5. Arrange remaining beads on a length of thread.
    6. Place your elbow on a table.
    7. Hold the thread so that the beads dangle.
    8. The large bead should swing easily without touching the table.
    9. Fold the thread at your fingertips.
    10. Loop the folded end around and through to create a knot.
    11. Pull tight.
    12. Cut off the remaining loose thread approximately ¼ inch from knot

To check the rotation of your pendulum:

- You can program the pendulum any way you like as long as the direction is always the same for the 'yes' or 'no' answer. E.g. Circle for 'yes', straight line for 'no'.
- Another way *(Hannah Kroeger's Way)* is to hold your hand flat on a table and draw your hand on paper.

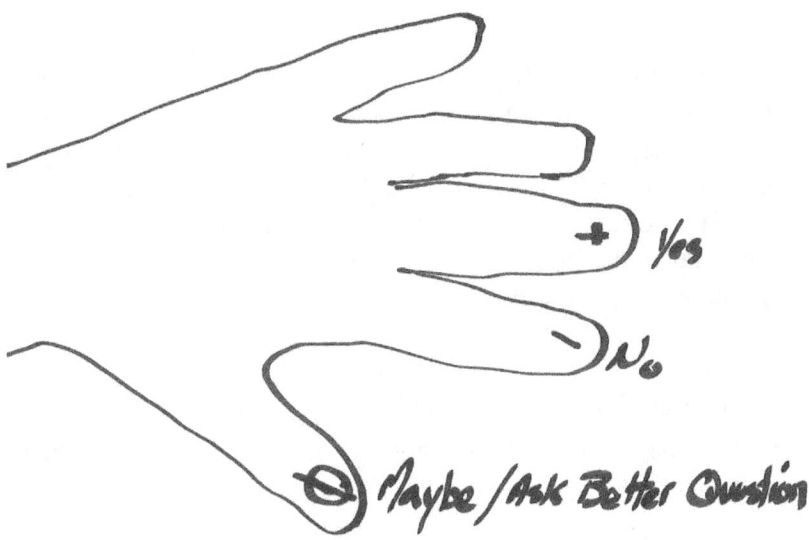

- Hold the pendulum over your middle fingernail; ask the pendulum to show you a 'yes' motion. Repeat until the pendulum <u>always</u> moves in the same direction, no matter if you stop and start. This finger is positive polarity.
- Next, move to the pointer fingernail; ask the pendulum to show you a 'no' motion. Repeat until the pendulum <u>always</u> moves in the same direction no matter if you stop and start. This finger is negative polarity.

- Hold the pendulum over your thumbnail; ask the pendulum to show you a 'neutral' or 'ask a better question' motion. Repeat until the pendulum <u>always</u> moves in the same direction no matter if you stop and start. This finger is a neutral polarity.

*Repeat this until you always have the same movements for each motion… to learn this it may take minutes, hours, days, weeks or months.

Your brain is like a highly developed computer, unconsciously knowing everything it has ever seen, heard, felt or thought since conception to now and, if you believe in past lives, that also. So, when we program our bodies to answer in a 'yes' or 'no' function, it will do just that. Every person has the answers to his/her own situation; he/she just needs to be shown how to ask the right questions.

Pendulum Exercise: (to receive a 'yes' or 'no' answer)

Always ask if you are "on" and if you can answer the questions. If yes:

- Have a person say his/her question out loud.
- Take a breath and clear your mind.
- Saying, "With integrity and honesty," then swing the pendulum.
- Answer the question.
- Repeat, until all questions are asked and answered.

(Sometimes I do this and another reading at the same time.)

TESTING METHOD #7:
Paper:

1) Write the word 'Yes' on a piece of paper about 2 inches x 2 inches.

2) Write the word 'No' on a piece of paper about 2 inches x 2 inches.

3) Have the person put one of the papers into each hand

4) Create a literal question and have the person mix up the papers (still one in each hand) and then you choose a hand.

5) We use this method a lot in our family, you cannot manipulate the answer **ever.** *When the answer has something to do with you, the mind can alter the answer when using the other methods.*

*Sometimes, we ask the question in our minds without saying the question out loud. *To make it even more fail proof, we have written the question down so no one can change what was asked.*

When you trust using the paper muscle testing method; you can also choose a 'yes / no' for each hand, as if you were holding a piece of paper (pretend) and answer the question.

***When I am Muscle Testing Answers for my client, I always ask myself:
- If I am on?
- Is my name Connie?

- Can I answer their questions?
    If the answer to all is 'Yes', I proceed.
- Then I say with honesty and integrity and answer the questions

**There are many ways to muscle test!
Whatever way works for you is the key.**

Practice, Practice, Practice!

THE SECRET IS... IN THE QUESTION

The trick is not the answer; the key is actually the question you ask! If you have not asked a literal question that is VERY specific, you may not actually understand the answer properly.

Example #1

If a man was bald walking down the street and you muscle tested if he had hair on his head, the answer probably will come back 'yes'. He has eyebrows, facial hair, etc. His head is literal from neck up.

Example #2

If you want to know if you can heal a person...

Question:

Can I <u>help</u> this person?
Can I <u>cure</u> this person?
Two very different questions

**The mind is just like a computer...
<u>very literal and focused</u>.
There are no slang words when asking yes, or no.**

EXAMPLE QUESTIONS

Your Intent / Thought #1 –
If I need to heal myself…

Question:

Where should I go to get help? Is there **someone** that can heal me?

Answer:

If Yes…

I always ask if I can heal myself first.

If No, then I ask, "Is there someone in Kelowna that can heal me"?

If No, then I ask, "Is there someone in the Okanagan that can heal me"?

If No, then I ask, "Is there someone in the British Columbia that can heal me"?

Then I go get a map and start by dividing the map into the upper and bottom sections and test.

Then do this again until I have a more detailed area, that I can ask for a city, then I go Google the practitioners of that area

If No…

Is there **something** that can heal me?

If Yes

Is it in my house…office…building…

Is it in this room? (muscle test until you have the room)

Then I divide the room…this side…this shelf…etc. until you find the specific item.

If you get 'No' to both questions, then at this moment in time there is nothing to heal you.

Your Intent / Thought #2 –
What vitamins to take…

Hold the container with the vitamin or supplement you would like to test

Question:

Should I take this _____ *(whatever you are holding)* today?

If No, try another if you would like to

If Yes

Test how many…1, 2, 3, etc.

When… now, morning, afternoon, dinner, bedtime…etc.

Your Intent / Thought #3 –
What book should I read...

In a bookstore

Question:

I 99% of the time test when I am in the bookstore if I should buy a book, and this book today?

If Yes

Test - is it in this section... *(most bookstores have signs showing what category you are in)*

Test – is it on this shelf?

Divide the shelf in your mind and test section

Then test which individual book

Is there another book to buy today?

Here?

Repeat if yes

If yes but not there, then you will have to muscle testing by asking more questions about where.

You can do this for any product anywhere you are!

Your Intent / Thought #4 –
Curing Rosacea…

Connie's 1st Story

I had a lady come in very upset, her Doctor had told her that she had Rosacea on her cheeks and that she would have it for the rest of her life. She was in her sixty's and quite beautiful, it devastated her that this pinky-red rash-like marks would be on her face for the rest of her life.
At the time that she came in, I did not know what Rosacea was, and I had to look the condition up in this book to read about the condition:

> '*Prescription for Nutritional Healing,* **Fifth Edition: A Practical A-to-Z Reference to Drug-Free Remedies Using Vitamins, Minerals, Herbs & Food A-To-Z Reference to Drug-Free Remedies Paperback – October 5, 2010,** *by* <u>**Phyllis A. Balch CNC**</u> **(Author)**

I taught her how to Muscle Test – Body Pendulum. I asked permission to Muscle Test her. She said, "Yes".

My client is sitting in my chair at my center

Question:

    I always test if I am on? Yes

    Is my name Connie? Yes

    Can I answer _____ (client's name) questions? Yes

    Can I cure her? No

    Is there something in my center that can cure her? Yes

Is it in this room? No

Is it in the front retail area? Yes (we go to the front area)

Is it a book? No

Is it a supplement/herb? Yes (I had three shelves full of products)

Is it in this column? No

Is it in this column? Yes (middle column had five shelves)

Is it these two top shelves? No

Is it on this shelf? No

Is it on this shelf? No

The bottom shelf had six different products on it…

Is it on this half? Yes (three products – I just picked up all three and gave her one at a time)

She muscle tested one at a time asking "is it this one that will cure my Rosacea…

It said yes to Apple Cider Vinegar

Then she muscle tested as I asked the questions…

Do you put it on your face? Yes

When? Morning

For how long? 1 Week

Are we done? No

Do you drink it? Yes

How much, capful? Yes

How often? Daily

For how long? 1 week

Are we done? No

It ended up that she needed to muscle test her make-up at home if she could use it?

Are we done? Yes

She came in three days later and showed me that her Rosacea was almost gone and that she tested, and she had to get rid of some of her make-up and change shampoo.

By the end of a week, the Rosacea was gone. I saw her three years later with her daughter in a store, and it had never come back.

Your Intent / Thought #5 –
Blessed Rice...

2nd Story

Years ago, when I had moved my business to the Dolphin road location, I use to have this man come in and test me. He would just show up and I was always fascinated with what he wanted to test, so I let him come.

Once he brought three containers of cooked rice, marked A, B & C. He said he blessed one, which one? Another time he brought a cut-up banana.

Question:

    Which container is holding the blessed rice?

    Container A? No

    Container B? No

    Container C? Yes

    Hey, it is possible that he did not bless any of them...I was correct.

Your Intent / Thought #6
– Blessed Banana
(same banana cut into three pieces)…

Question:

    Which bag is holding the blessed piece of banana?

    Bag A? No

    Bag B? No

    Bag C? No

He said that for sure one is blessed... I thought about it for a moment and remembered that the peel of a banana is poisonous and asked him to take off the peel of each and but back in the appropriate bag. He did.

Question:

    Which bag is holding the blessed piece of peeled banana?

    Bag A? No

    Bag B? Yes

    Bag C? No

    I was correct

Your Intent / Thought #7 –
Cure Hepatitis C…

3rd Story

I had the husband of a client come in and we muscle tested if I could cure him. He had caught Hepatitis C.

Question:

    I always test if I am on? Yes

    Is my name Connie? Yes

    Can I answer _____ (client's name) questions? Yes

    Can I cure him? No

    Can he cure himself? Yes

    Is it something I know how to do? Yes… It muscle tested Hypnotherapy

It ended up being a story of him draining his motorcycle engine a metaphor to his liver.

He came back three months later and told me his Hepatitis C was cured.

I did not cure him; he did, by repeating the story in his mind every day.

Your Intent / Thought#8 –
Cure Back Pain...

4th Story

In the first few months that I had learned Muscle Testing, my Mom called me to ask if I could see one of her friends really quick. He and his wife were going to drive back home (two-day trip) and his back was out.

Question:

    I always test if I am on? Yes

    Is my name Connie? Yes

    Can I answer _____ (client's name) questions? Yes

    Can I cure him? Yes

    How, by the quick-fix method? Yes

We did the quick fix method two times and I remember him saying, "Is that all."

"Yep, that is it." I replied.

My Mom told me a few days later he called and told her that he was amazed that he felt better instantly and the pain never came back. The Muscle Testing Quick Fix is in the 'How To Balance Your Muscles' portion. I show my clients this method to almost anyone in pain that wants to be able to look after themselves.

Pain seems to be an easy one to cure by using these muscle testing techniques, if the pain does not change then it is usually a bone issue (Need a Chiropractor).

Your Intent / Thought #9 –
My Daughters question that she wrote down...

5th Story

When my children where teenagers, especially my daughter, would ask me if he/she could go out to a party or something else that was equally as hard to answer.

Question:

    I always test if I am on? Yes

    Is my name Connie? Yes

    Can I answer _____ (my daughter's) questions? Yes

    She thinks the question that she has written down on the paper, and I answer... Saying to myself, "Honesty and with integrity."

    Then tested for yes or no

Amazingly enough, she received the answer she wanted more than I consciously would have said okay to. Before learning muscle testing; she would ask to go to a party or something and my natural instinct was to instantly say no.

All I cared about was her safety...I guess God knows better than I did...

Muscle Testing really made life easy for me with teenagers, *because the rule was whatever the answer was, we all of us had to follow.*

WHAT CAN YOU MUSCLE TEST FOR?

Anything you need an answer to.
What if my muscle testing is not answering at all?

> Sometimes it can be the wrong time to ask the question, or the question is not specific enough, or you need to go pee first (a full bladder is hard for the brain to hold and answer questions), or you may need to drink some water to hydrate.

Will Muscle Testing work for personal questions?

> Yes, but remember sometimes when it is about you, you can manipulate the answer.
>
> You may want to ask if you can ask and get an honest answer first.
>
> I like to use the paper method.

Can I ask questions about other people?

> Only if it is your child (and they are under the legal age) or you are their guardian.
>
> Morally you need the person's permission to get honest answers.
>
> *I imagine it is like breaking into a person's house and going through their belongings or filing cabinet...only a*

dishonest person would do that.

Can I ask questions about my pets?

> Yes, you are their guardian

Can I ask the winning lotto numbers?

> Sure, but ask if you will win
>
> What winning numbers are they for – what lotto ticket? And for where – city, state, country? And for what date? Soooo many questions to ask to get the perfect timing for something like that…Good luck though!

What do I use Muscle Testing for?

- To get answers for my clients
- To get personal answers for me
- To decide what vitamins to take and how many
- To choose which item to buy when I am unsure
- Any decision that my husband and I cannot agree on
- How to heal me
- If I can or cannot do something

How often can I test?

> In the beginning, you may start to test everything, and it is good to practice. Once you get the hang of it, you will only test when you have a dilemma or if another person has a question.

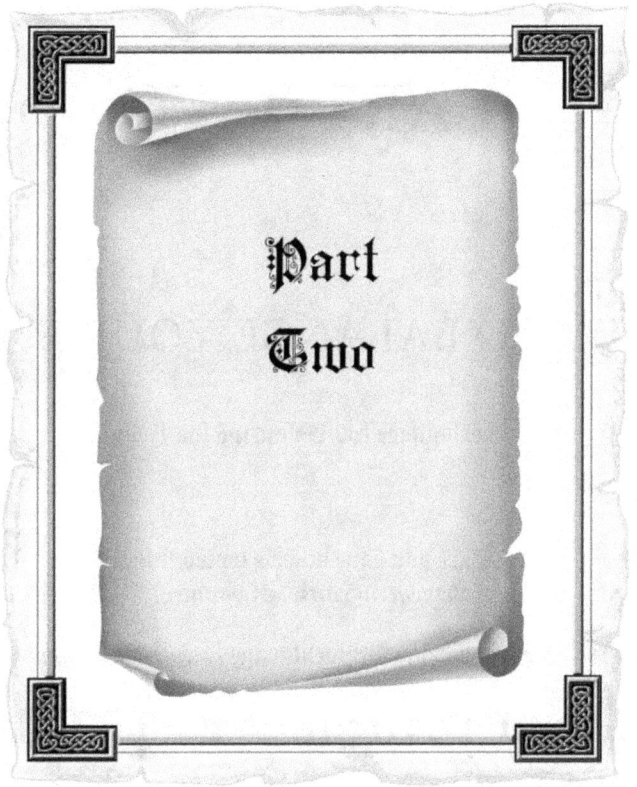

Part Two

PART TWO

HOW TO BALANCE YOUR BODY

Techniques for Balancing the Body

Once you have muscle tested if the element/organ is off balance...

The following are many different ways to balance the *meridians*.

Find Your Favorite Way To Balance.

BONUS
Exercise to Practice

Movement Activity – AKA Cross Crawl

This activity integrates the two hemispheres (left and right sides) of the brain simultaneously. Moving the opposite arms and legs together encourages concentration, moves the lymph and stimulates coordination, energy, and ability to focus. This is a wonderful activity to prepare for sports, exercise, and dance. It also boosts concentration, alertness, and creativity.

It has been said that a child who does not learn to crawl before walking does not develop both sides of the brain hemisphere as well as a child who does crawl. Studies have shown that a child who crawls is more developed. We can retrain the brain at any age.

Movement – use any movement that creates opposite arm and leg movements, for example, left elbow to right knee (bring a bent knee up). Ensure that the arms swing freely from the shoulders and that the elbows bend. The head should remain neutral. Enhance the activity with music that encourages this movement.

You may also introduce left hand to right heel and switch to the opposite hand and heel, behind you.

Do this routine as many times as needed – (muscle test how many times).

BALANCING METHOD #1
Quick Fix

My Favorite!

You can do this sitting or standing. You usually do this on your body to show him where to touch, while the person does it simultaneously on his own. Say,

"In just a few moments you are going to rub some points on your body. First, take a breath and sense if there is any pain or discomfort anywhere in your body. Put a number to it, 1 being hardly any problem and 10 being almost unbearable… "

This is very important since most people need some kind of comparison to determine if anything worked.

<u>Starting with the front of your body:</u>

1) Using your thumb and middle finger (left or right-hand does not matter), or using both pointer fingers, place the two fingers just below your collar bone and about two inches on either side of your breastbone (letter B). You should feel or notice an indentation on either side that might be sensitive or painful. Lightly rub in either direction (some people believe it has to be in a clockwise direction, but I have found it works either way). Do this for a few moments. Make sure you keep breathing.

2) Next, with the karate chop part of your hand (ulna side) or your fingertips, rub up and down (distance is approximately four to five inches) just on the outside (lateral) of the breast, not quite under the arm (letter A), three to five times. You can do both sides of the body simultaneously or one at a time.

3) With your fingertips, you will now rub up and down your sternum (between your breasts, letters J, E, M & K). Most of

these movements I do three to five times on each point. You can do more if you like.

4) I use my thumbs next; rub just under the breast area on your ribs (letter L & C). I start in the middle and go outwards.

5) Next follow along with your diaphragm, the bottom of your rib cage (letter F) in the same motion as before.

6) Now imagine you have four corners around your belly button and rub/press all four at once (G & H).

7) With either hand, using the karate chop part (ulna side), touch your body between your hips, just above the pubic bone and rub from left to right a few times (letter I & G).

8) Using the palms of your hands, rub the outside of both legs downwards to your knees (letter N & I), three to five times.

9) Now follow the same procedure on the inside of your legs (Letter N& F).

Now the focus is on the back of your body:

10) Using your pointer fingers, rub 'A, Ren' on the back of the neck. Bend the head slightly forward, rub the indents on either side of the spine just below the skull (Cervical 1, Cervical 2)

11) Using either a corner of a doorway or your hand (if you can reach), rub your spinal column from about your shoulder blades all the way down to your hips (letter B, E, J, M, K, L, C, D, F, H), again two or three times.

12) Now, on either side of your spine, rub the yellow triangles (letter N, G & I) up and down.

13) Using the opposite hand, starting at the outside of the shoulder, lightly pinch along the top of your shoulder towards the ear (xxxxxx– letter O), two to three times.

13) Now take a couple of deep breaths and <u>re-evaluate</u> the pain level or number at which you started. Most people find that the pain is gone completely with just doing this once.

-Repeat a second time if the number did not go to a zero.

-If, after a second time, the number has not gone to a zero, you may need to go to a chiropractor for an adjustment. I have also had a client who had pain in a bone in his foot that had not healed, and the body was protecting itself from injury. So be careful to give yourself time to heal if you have hurt yourself.

> *I had been working in the industrial sewing business since I was twelve as my parents owned an awning and manufacturing business. After fourteen years of sewing in both my parents and then my own company, and two children later, my back went out. I never really knew what would precipitate the pain. All I seemed to have to do was just pick up a pencil from the ground and it would go out so badly that I would end up on the floor from the sheer pain and without help, could not move for days.*
>
> *This had been going on for about two years and only the chiropractor was able to keep it in place, but it always seemed to go out on the weekends when he wasn't working. The diagnosis was that my spine could no longer tolerate all those years of repetitive motion and that I had no stomach muscles. And, to boot, the x-rays showed that I had one extra vertebra in the lumbar part of my lower back.*
>
> *I sold my business in the hope that it would solve the problem, but the difficulties continued. An operation was to be my last resort. This idea didn't thrill me too much, so I decided to try alternative medicine. I started taking classes on Muscle Testing where I learned this*

method of balancing. I personally had to do this exercise two to three times a day for months and at least once a day for a year until my body retrained itself and the muscles grew back to their proper position.

Who would have thought that something so simple that anyone could do, once learned, would mean no cost and no more pain?

The great thing is I didn't need that operation after all, and my back is still fine. It was many years later before I had to see the chiropractor again and this time it was because my sciatic nerve started to make me take notice for, I wasn't getting enough exercise.

A client of mine did the original drawing of this chart for me way back in 1999...

Muscle Testing - Quick Fix

1) Ask client to sense his body's area(s) of pain. On a scale of 1-10, 10 being major pain, ask the client to tell you his level.
2) Lightly rub or have client rub all the front and back Neuro-lymphatic points.
3) Have client take a deep breath and re-sense his level of pain.
4) If the pain has not come down to 0, redo the "quick fix" sequence.
5) If pain level does not come to 0 the second time, the client may need to have a chiropractic adjustment or need a different type of treatment, or you may try to relax/quiet individual muscles.

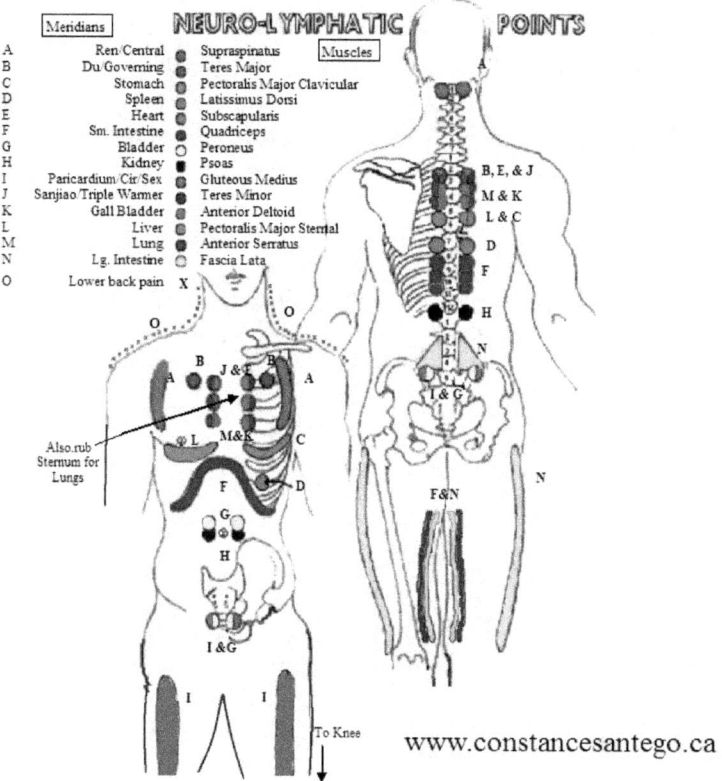

BALANCING METHOD #2
Meridian Walking

This procedure balances the energy in a meridian

This may be easiest to accomplish when the person is lying down.

" After determining which meridians need balancing:

" Start at both the first and last point on the meridian by lightly holding your finger on both tsubo point.

" Take notice of which one of your fingers starts to tingle or have hot or cold sensations first and then move that finger only to the next point on the meridian in the direction of the other hand.

" When your fingers meet on the meridian rub the tsubo in the correct direction (kyo or jitsu).

" When completed all meridians recheck the level of pain on a scale of 0 - 10.

BALANCING METHOD #3
Source Points

- ➢ Another term for source point is 'balancing point'.
- ➢ Source points are stationed on the meridian they control.
- ➢ Located on the hands and feet (opposite for left & right).
- ➢ Source point = Main Tsubo to balance the entire meridian.

Procedure: With medium pressure hold the source point for thirty seconds to one minute.

For a Full Body Balance Hold: Ren – BL 10 & Du - KI 27

Individual:
Dorsal side of wrist
LI 4, SJ 4 & SI 4

Palm side of wrist
HT 7, LU 9 & PC 7

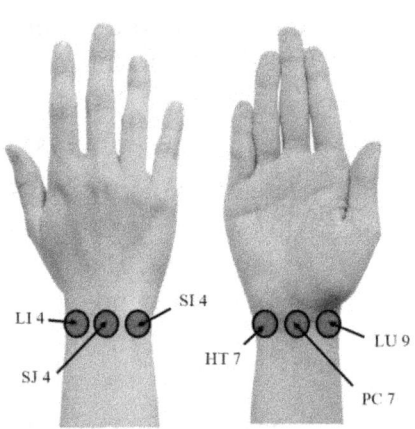

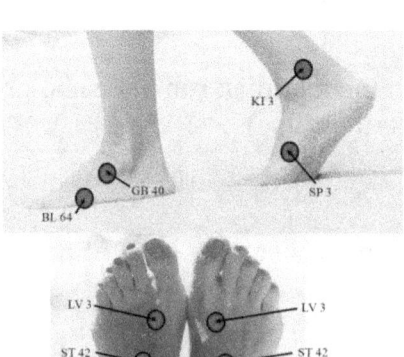

Lateral side of foot
GB 40 & BL 64

Medial side of foot
KI 3 & SP 3

Dorsal side of foot
St 42 & LV 3

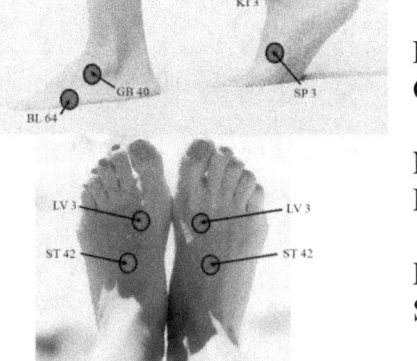

BALANCING METHOD #4
Strengthen / Weaken

Balancing Method #5 - Strengthening or Weakening the Muscle

On the next 14 pages you will find the origin and insertion of each muscle.

Find the belly of the muscle. (In the direction of the muscle fiber, the belly is the center between the origin and insertion points.)

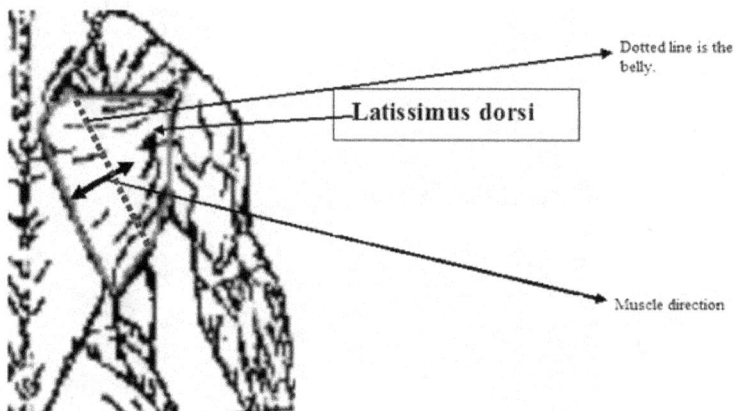

Once you have located the belly, muscle test the client to find out if that muscle is deficient/depleted or in excess (this procedure is a little different than Kyo or Jitsu).

one
-If the muscle test is <u>excessive,</u> move your fingers (pointer and thumb) across the belly (from side to the other). Fingers start *apart* and *move together* (like you would do a pinch, but you do not pinch them really, it is just the motion).

-If the muscle test is <u>deficient/depleted</u>, move your fingers (pointer and thumb) across the belly (from one side to the other). Fingers start *together* and *move apart* (opposite movement to excess).

Lung Meridian (LU)
Points: 11
Sign: Yin

Lung Meridian
The Liver meridian at the outer portion of the chest where the clavicle meets the humerus. It travels along the insides of the arms to the outside base of the thumbnail.

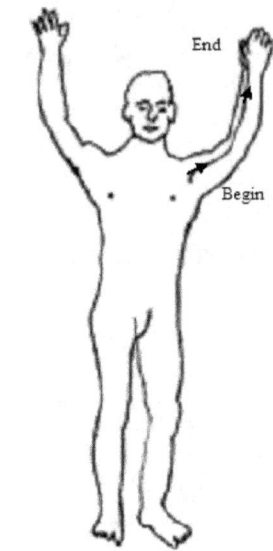

Anterior Serratus
The serratus muscle draws the shoulder blade forward and raises the ribs.

Origin:
The outer surface of the upper 9 ribs on the side of the chest.

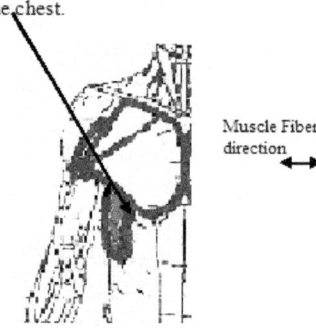

Muscle Fiber direction

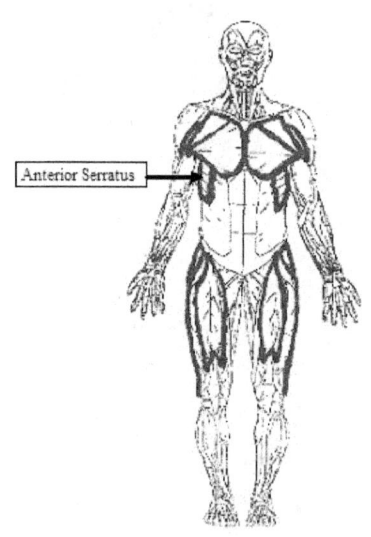

Anterior Serratus

Insertion:
On the inner surface of the scapula, along the edge nearest to the spine. (This muscle wraps around the body to the back of the body.)

Large Intestine Meridian (LI)
Points: 20
Sign: Yang

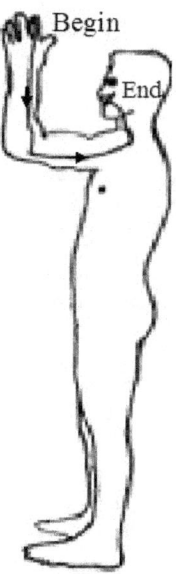

Large Intestine Meridian
The large intestine meridian begins at the base of the index finger and runs up the outside of the hand and arms. It crosses over the shoulder, up the throat and over the jaw to the side of the nose.

Fascia Latae
This fascia latae is a muscle / tendon which helps to flex or bend the thigh, draw it away from the body sideways, and keep it turned in.

Origin:
On the edge of the anterior portion of the hip bone.

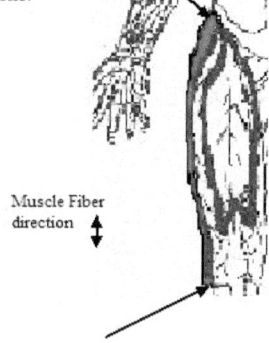

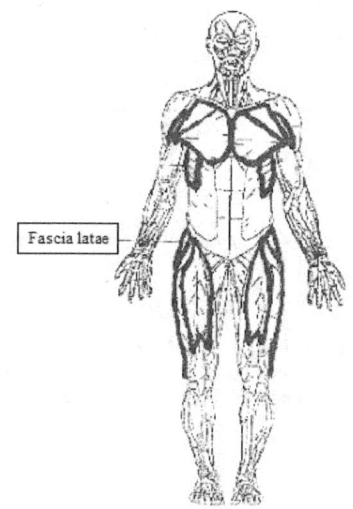

Insertion:
Just below the knee on the outside of the leg.

Stomach meridian (ST)
Points: 45
Sign: Yang

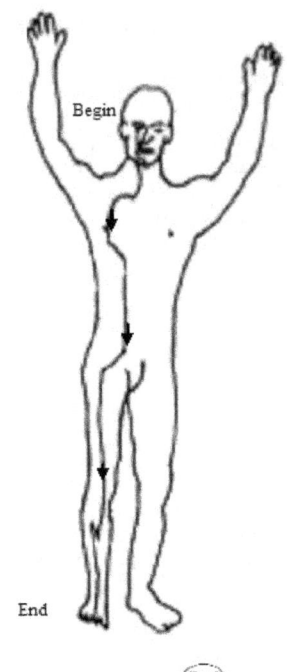

Stomach Meridian
The stomach meridian begins below the center of the eyes. It descends down the sides of the throat, through the chest, nipples, abdomen, and groin, where it jogs over to and goes down the outside of the legs, over the instep, ending at the base of the second toenail

Pectoralis major clavicular
The chest muscle helps bend and turn the arm at the shoulder.

Origin:
Middle of the collar bone to the knob on the inner end at the base of the throat.

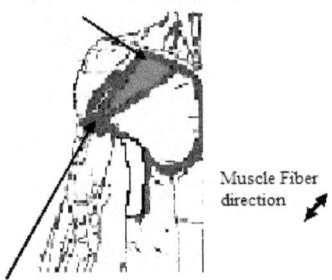

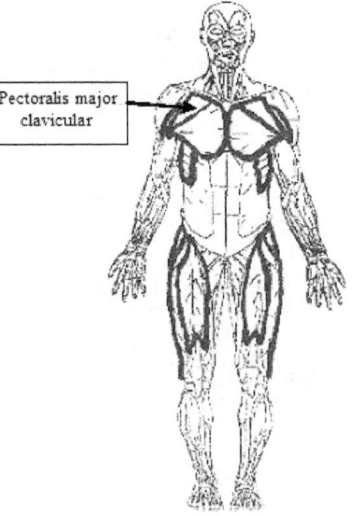

Insertion:
The groove between the muscles at the front of the upper arm, just below the shoulder.

Spleen Meridian (SP)
Points: 21
Sign: Yin

Spleen Meridian
The spleen meridian begins at the base of the large toenail. It travels up the insides of the leg to the groin, through the abdominal cavity, up over the ribs, underneath the armpits.

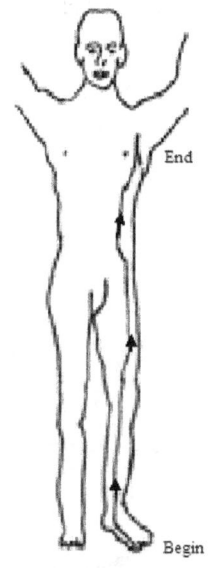

Latissimus Dorsi
The muscle holds the shoulder down and helps keep the back straight.

Origin:
Along the spine from between the lower part of the shoulder blades down to the level of the hips.

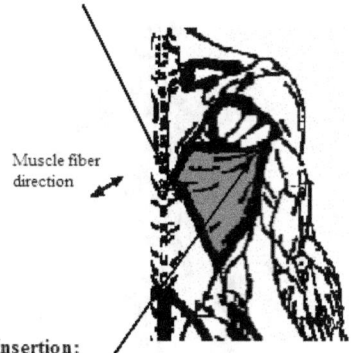

Insertion:
Inside of the arm just below the shoulder.

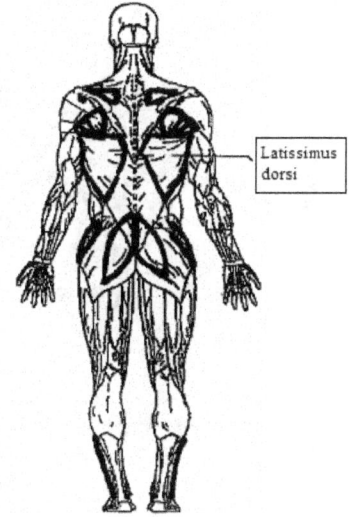

Heart Meridian (HT)
Points: 9
Sign: Yin

Heart Meridian
The heart meridian begins in the center of the armpit and moves along the inside of the arm to the inside base of the little fingernail.

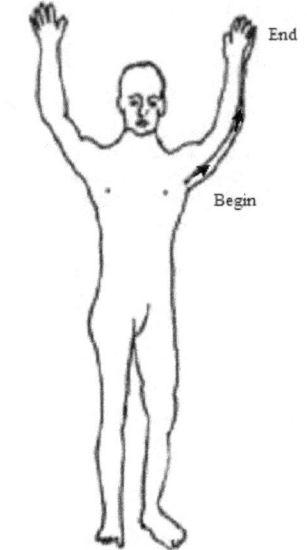

Subscapularis
The subscapularis cannot be seen or felt because it is behind the scapula. It allows the shoulder blade to glide over the rib cage and turn the arm, drawing the arm in when it is raised above the shoulder.

Origin:
Inner surface of the shoulder blade.

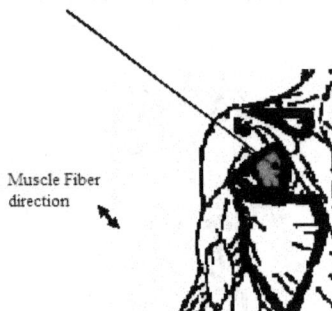

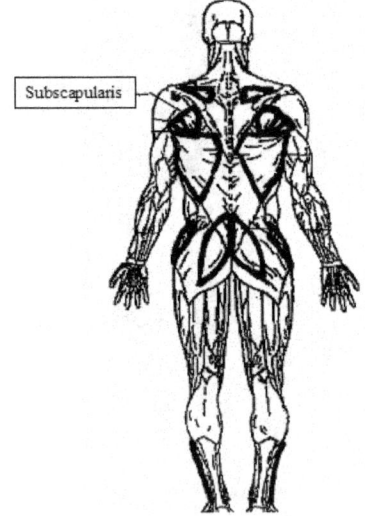

Insertion:
In front of the top of the humerus (front of body).

Small Intestine Meridian (SI)
Points: 20
Sign: Yang

Small Intestine Meridian
The small intestine meridian begins at the base of the little finger. It moves along the outer arm to the shoulder. Then it zigzags through the scapula, travels up and over the shoulder to the base of the neck and ends on the face in front of the ear.

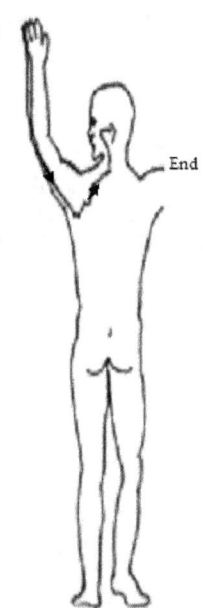

Quadriceps
This muscle straightens the knee and flexes the thigh.

Origin:
Upper portion of the femur and the side of the hip bone.

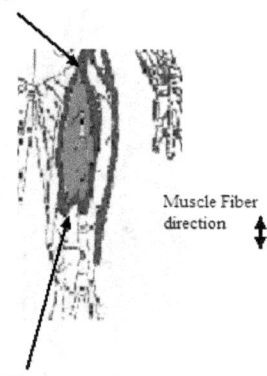

Insertion:
On the shinbone, just below the knee cap.

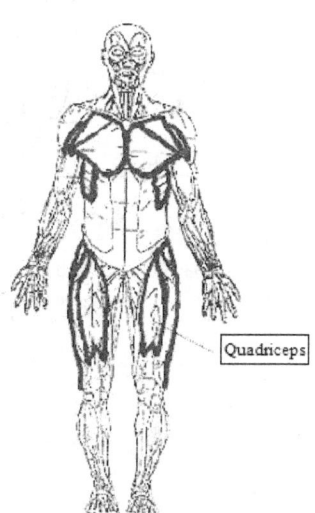

Bladder Meridian (BL)
Points: 67
Sign: Yang

Bladder Meridian
The bladder meridian begins at the inside corner of the eyes, moves over the skull, down each side of the spine, down the back of the legs, to the outside base of the little toenail.

Peroneus
The peroneus muscle flexes the side of the foot upward and out.

Origin:
Outer side of the lower leg.

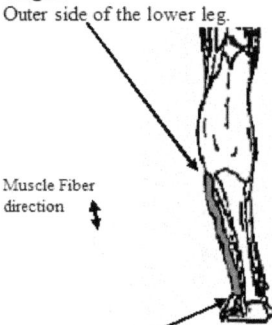

Muscle Fiber direction

Insertion:
Outer side of the foot and across the arch on top of the foot.

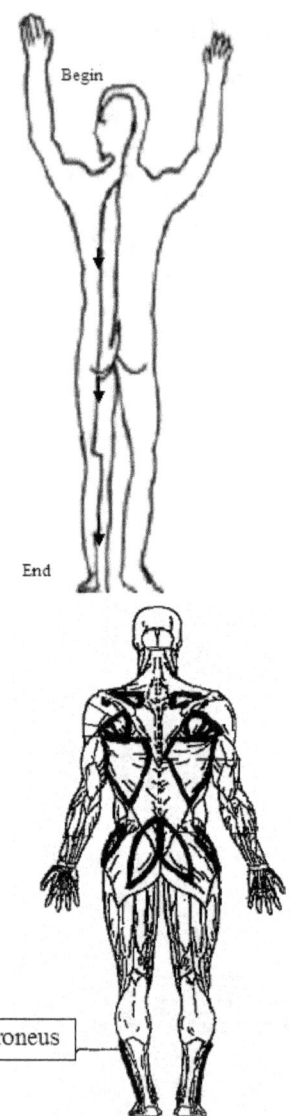

Kidney Meridian (KI)
Points: 27
Sign: Yin

Kidney Meridian
The kidney meridian begins at the soles of the feet, and runs up the innermost part of the leg, to the genital region. It runs from the pubic bone, up the abdomen near the midline, to end in the indentations just below the clavicle.

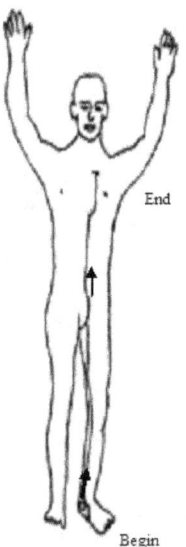

Psoas
This muscle is part of the hip flexors. It helps keep the lumbar curve in the spine.

Origin:
Along the spine from T12, the level of the last rib, and all the lumbar vertebrae.

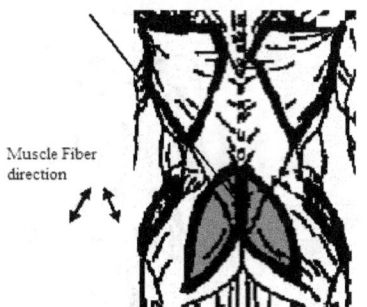

Muscle Fiber direction

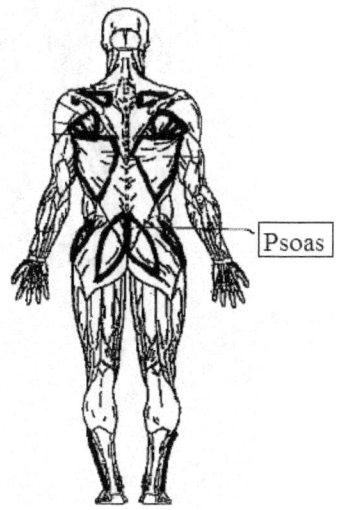

Insertion:
Inside of the upper part of the thigh bone, about level with the pubic bone (front side of the body).

Pericardium or Circulation/Sex Meridian
Points: 20
Sign: Yin

Pericardium or Circulation/Sex Meridian
The circulation-sex meridian runs from the outside of the nipple along the biceps muscle, through the inside of the arm to the tip of the middle finger.

Gluteus Medius
The gluteus medius is used to pull the thigh out and rotate the leg.

Origin:
Outer surface of the hip bone.

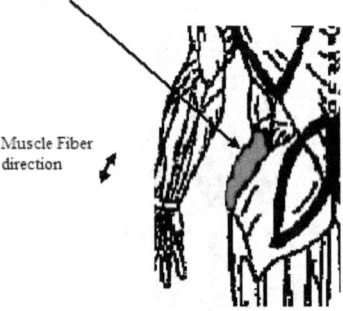

Insertion:
Top of the thigh bone at the side (comes around to the front of the body).

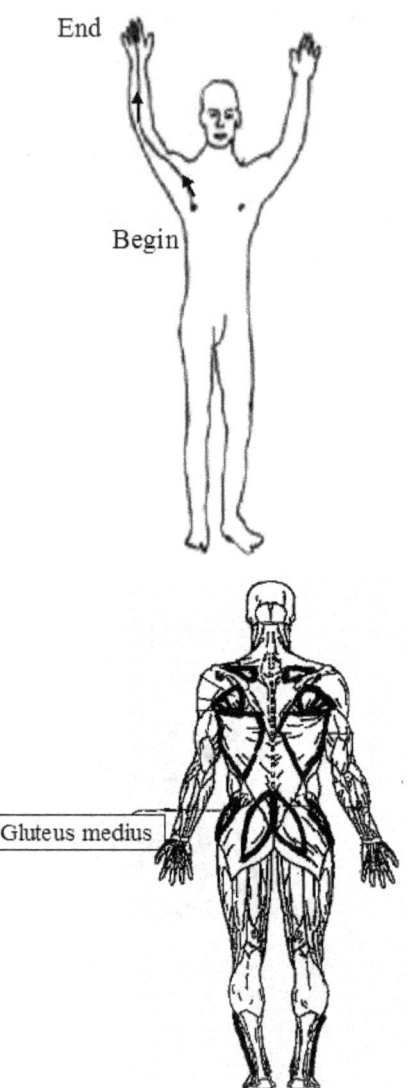

Sanjiao or
Triple Warmer Meridian
Points: 23
Sign: Yang
Endocrine system (Thyroid, adrenal and pituitary)

Sanjiao or Triple Warmer Meridian
The triple warmer meridian begins at the ring finger, runs along the back of the arm, around the shoulders, up the outside of the neck, and around the ear to the temples.

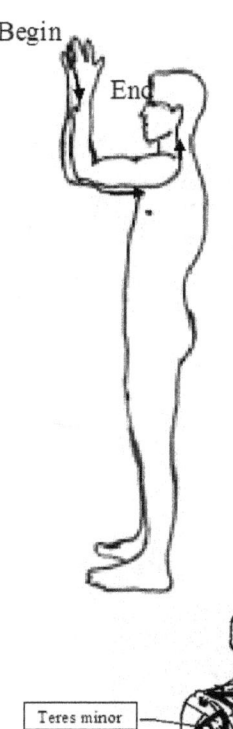

Teres Minor
This shoulder muscle rotates the arm and forearm.

Origin:
The edge of the shoulder blade closest to the spine.

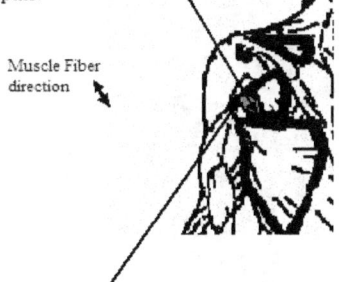

Muscle Fiber direction

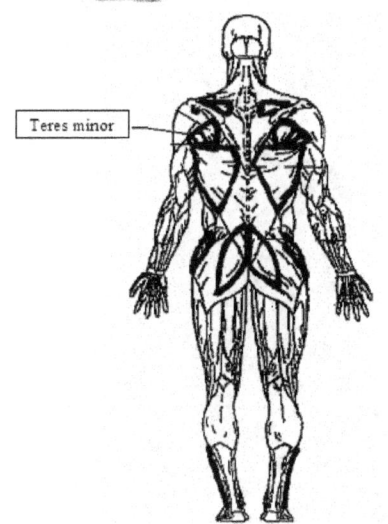

Teres minor

Insertion:
Top of the upper arm in the back.

Gall Bladder Meridian (GB)
Points: 44
Sign: Yang

Gall Bladder Meridian
The gall bladder meridian begins at the outer corner of the eyes. It zigzags over the sides of the skull and down the back of the neck and shoulders to the sides of the body. It then zigzags down the sides of the trunk to the outside of the hips, and runs down the legs to the end of the fourth toe.

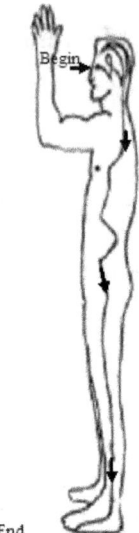

Anterior Deltoid
The anterior deltoid muscle is used when flexing the shoulder with the elbow bent. We use this muscle when we comb our hair.

Origin:
The outer third of the collar bone closest to the shoulder.

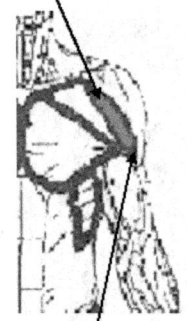

Muscle Fiber direction

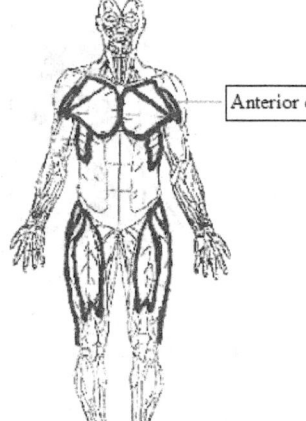

Insertion:
On the side of the arm about 1/3 down from the top of the humerus to the elbow.

Liver Meridian (LR)
Points: 20
Sign: Yin

Liver Meridian
The liver meridian begins at the inside base of the large toe. It runs up the inside of the leg and thigh, through the male and female reproductive organs, and underneath the rib cage into the Liver.

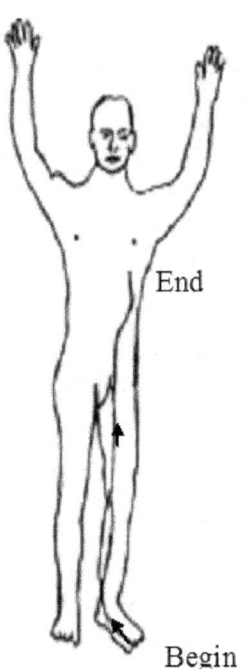
End

Begin

Pectoralis Major Sternal
The muscle is used when moving the arm in, and turning and drawing it forward.

Origin:
Along the sternum on the 4th to 7th ribs.

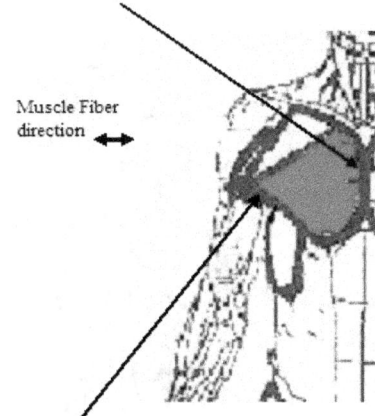

Muscle Fiber direction

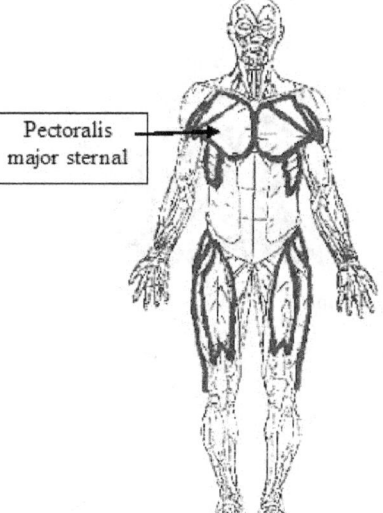

Pectoralis major sternal

Insertion:
The indentation between the muscles at the front of the upper arm.

Ren Meridian (RN) BL 10
AKA: Conception Vessel or Central
Points: 24
Sign: Yin

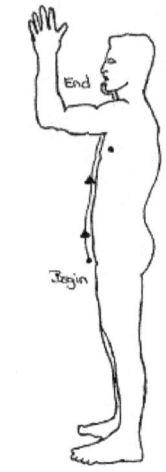

Ren Meridian
The Ren meridian flows from the center of the pubic bone (located between the scrotum and the anus in men, and between the posterior commissure of the labia and the anus in women), up the center of the body, under the chin to just below the lower lip.

Supraspinatus
This muscle helps in moving the arm away from the body and in holding the arm in the shoulder socket.

Origin:
Top, inner edge of the shoulder blade.

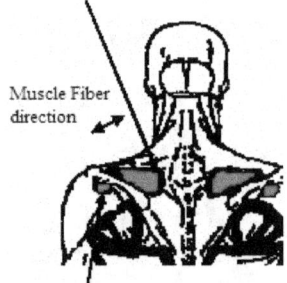

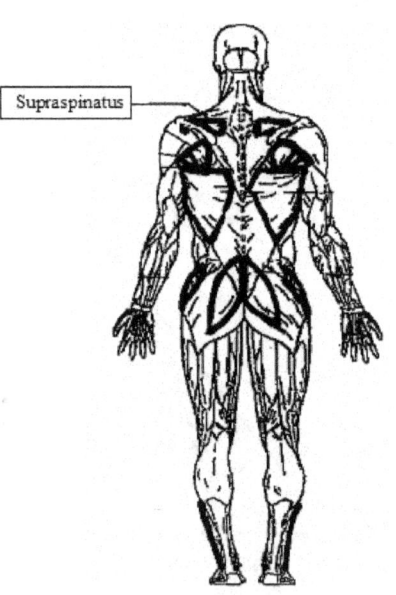

Insertion:
Top of the humerus.

Du Meridian (Du) K27 or RN21
AKA: Governing Vessel or Governing
Points: 28
Sign: Yang

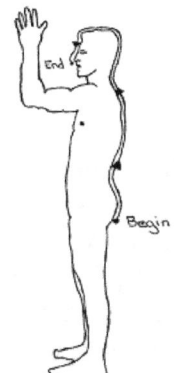

Du Meridian
The Du meridian flows from the perineum, up the spinal column, and over the head to the center of the upper lip.

Teres Major
This muscle in the back of the shoulder draws the arm in and keeps it turned out.

Origin:
Bottom corner of the shoulder blade.

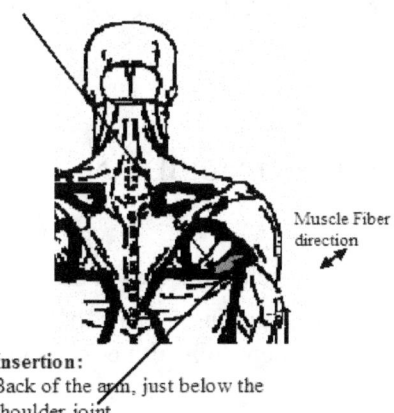

Muscle Fiber direction

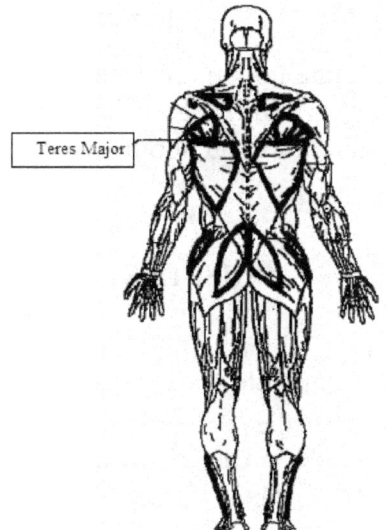

Teres Major

Insertion:
Back of the arm, just below the shoulder joint.

BALANCING METHOD #5
Muscles Massage

A Massage can also tell you what is going on in the body.

If you know how to do Swedish massage, then all you are doing is writing down which muscles are hypertonic, painful, hot, cold or weak. Muscles correspond to the meridians and organs of the body. Massage is another way to balance the meridians.

After you have written down which muscles the person is having issues with, then you will check if it corresponds to the muscles on the anterior, posterior or lateral meridian channels.

Notice how many muscles are corresponding to each body organ and if it correlates to the person's health form, issues they have told you about.

MUSCLES RELATED TO EACH MERIDIAN

If a muscle has an issue (hot, cold, hypertonicity muscle - tone /tight), then you can refer to which Meridian/Organ controls that muscle and determine if there are any coincident to health conditions in the body.

Point is to balance the muscle (relax or strengthen). Swedish Massage is an excellent technique to achieve the desired result.

SECRETS OF A HEALER – MAGIC OF MUSCLE TESTING

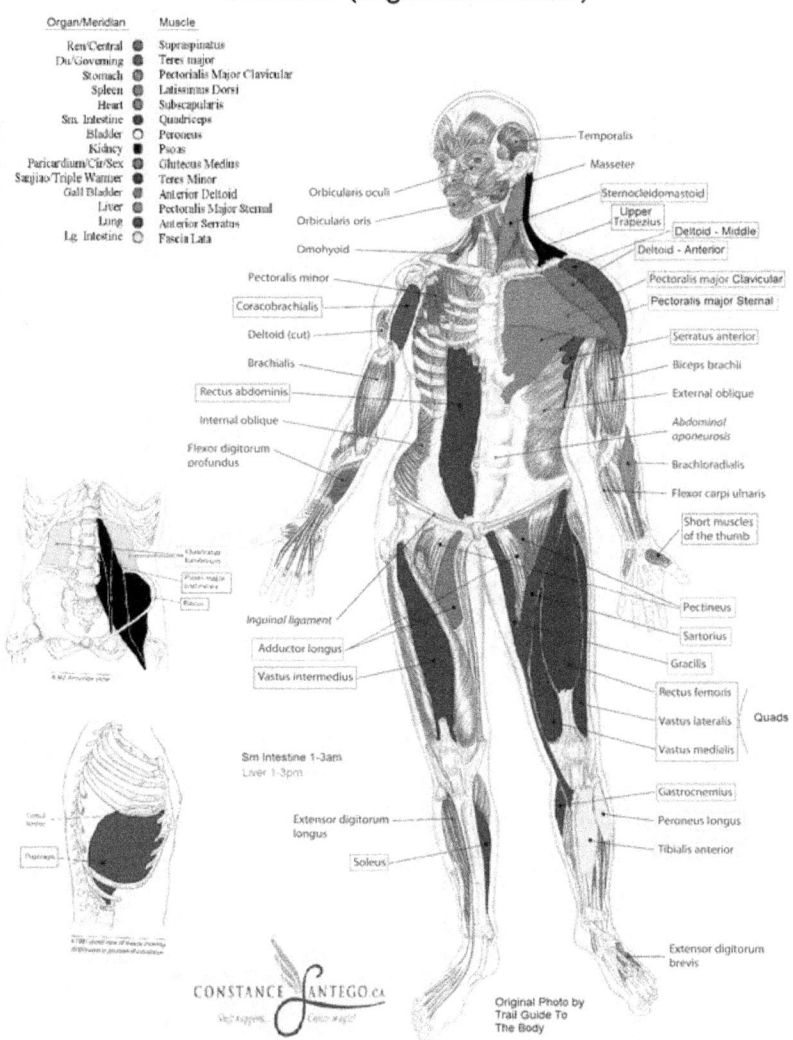

Muscles (organs/meridians)

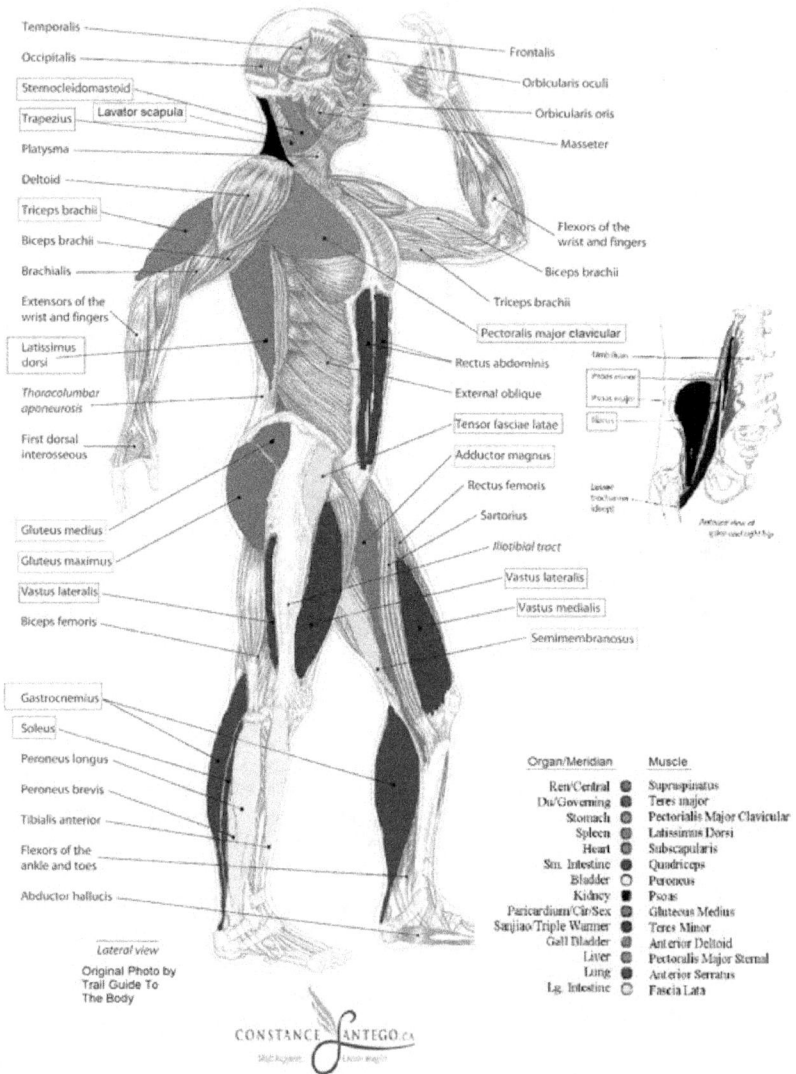

Lateral view
Original Photo by Trail Guide To The Body

Organ/Meridian	Muscle
Ren/Central	Supraspinatus
Du/Governing	Teres major
Stomach	Pectoralis Major Clavicular
Spleen	Latissimus Dorsi
Heart	Subscapularis
Sm. Intestine	Quadriceps
Bladder	Peroneus
Kidney	Psoas
Pericardium/Cir/Sex	Gluteus Medius
Sanjiao/Triple Warmer	Teres Minor
Gall Bladder	Anterior Deltoid
Liver	Pectoralis Major Sternal
Lung	Anterior Serratus
Lg. Intestine	Fascia Lata

Muscles (organs/meridians)

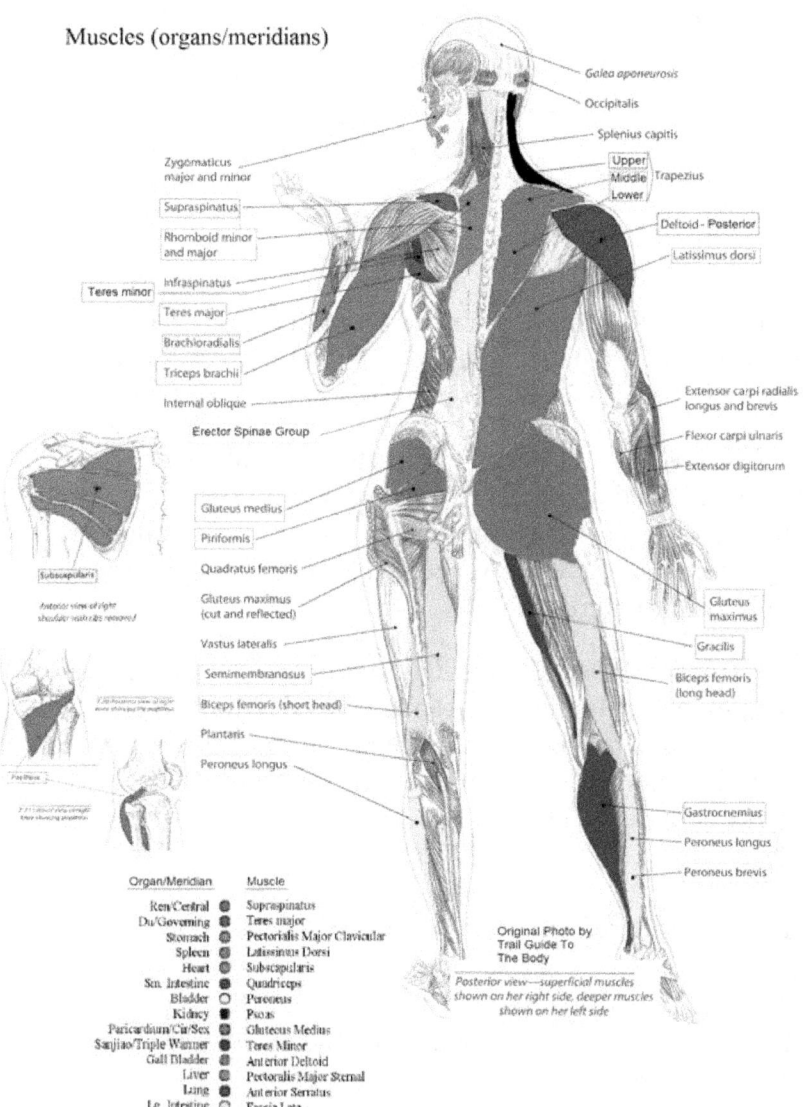

Organ/Meridian	Muscle
Ren/Central	Supraspinatus
Du/Governing	Teres major
Stomach	Pectoralis Major Clavicular
Spleen	Latissimus Dorsi
Heart	Subscapularis
Sm. Intestine	Quadriceps
Bladder	Peroneus
Kidney	Psoas
Pericardium/Cir/Sex	Gluteus Medius
Sanjiao/Triple Warmer	Teres Minor
Gall Bladder	Anterior Deltoid
Liver	Pectoralis Major Sternal
Lung	Anterior Serratus
Lg. Intestine	Fascia Lata

Original Photo by Trail Guide To The Body

Posterior view—superficial muscles shown on her right side, deeper muscles shown on her left side

BALANCING METHOD #6
Five Element Theory

THE PURPOSE OF THE FIVE ELEMENT CYCLE

Is to have a guide to use when determining what element (organ) is out of balance and then, with the use of the answers you found, bring balance/homeostasis back to the body.

It is thought that the Tsou Yen was the official creator of the doctrine of the five elements. The Nei Ching states, "The five elements - wood, fire, earth, metal, and water - encompass all the phenomena of nature. It is a symbolism that applies itself equally well to humankind."

These five symbols were created to reflect our experiences back to us. Some explain the five elements as five movements or phases. Each is related to a different season of the year which, in turn, is connected to an organ in the human body. By understanding each element, we can balance the dis-ease in the body.

Fire is considered summer—abundance, and action on the ideas.

Earth is considered late summer or Indian summer—harvest, reap our rewards.

Metal is considered fall or autumn—decline or withdrawal.

Water is considered winter—dormancy or hibernation.

Wood is considered spring—activity and new growth, ideas or beginnings.

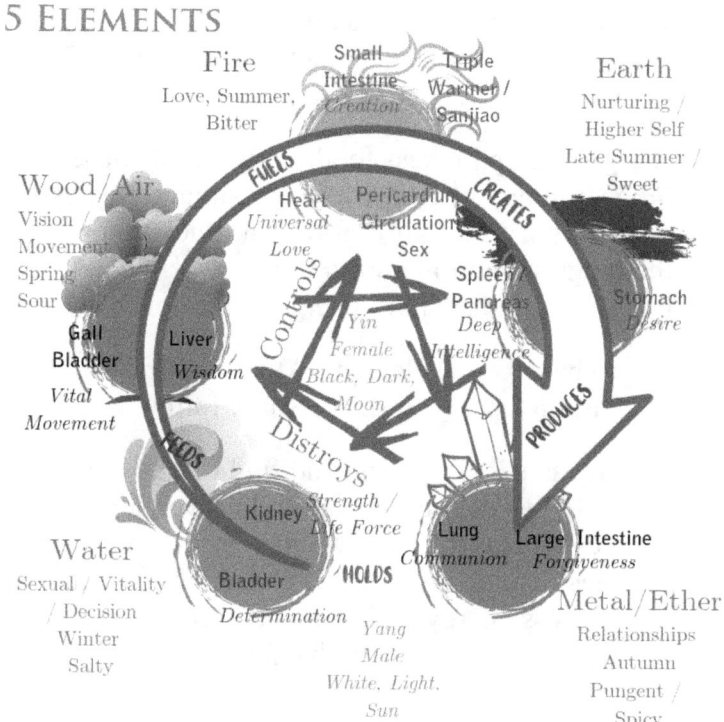

NOURISHING CYCLE

As you go <u>clockwise</u> around the five-element cycle picture (on the next page, you will find that each element helps the next one. Wood feeds the fire (burning the wood), fire makes earth (ashes turn into dirt), earth creates metal (iron and silver, for example, come from the earth), metal holds water (can be made into cups or enrich the water with mineral ores), water nourishes wood (creates it to grow).

> * **Water** element - **kidney** (yin organ) helps to feed the **wood** element - **liver** (yin organ) and strengthens its

energy. The liver generates blood, which is needed by the *fire* element - *heart* (yin organ) and strengthens its energy. The fiery energy of the heart supports the **earth** element - *spleen* (yin organ) and strengthens its energy. The spleen, by supplying the needed heat and

energy to help process food, nurtures the **metal** element - *lungs* (yin organ) by taking the resultant food essence and combines with the air to form chi. Back to the beginning, the lungs support the **water** element - *kidneys* (yin organ) by sending moist chi or energy to be stored in the kidneys.

One way to balance the element: After marking the five-element chart on a paper or the person's form.

When you muscle test a person and find that an element is deficient or depleted, you will check the five-element nourishing cycle chart and see what element is directly behind it and then boost that element (make it stronger/feed it/nourish it) so that the excess energy will bring balance back to the element that was low by overflowing with energy.

NOURISHING CYCLE

Wood feeds Fire

Fire makes Earth

Earth creates Metal

Metal holds Water

Water nurtures Wood

Nourishing

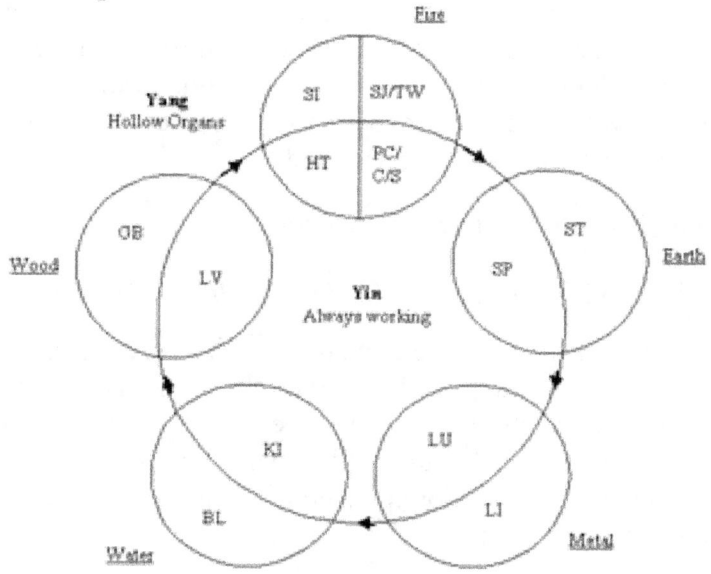

CONTROLLING CYCLE

Each element also can control or dominate another element. Imagine a five-pointed star in the middle of the chart. Wood consumes (depletes, grows and covers) earth, earth dams (absorbs) water, water extinguishes (overcomes) fire, fire melts metal, metal cuts (chopping it) wood.

A second way to balance the element:

After marking the five-element chart on the person's form.

When you muscle test a person and find that an element/organ is low in energy or depleted, you will check the five-element controlling cycle chart and see what element is across from it (follow the arrow backward) in the five-pointed star. This will show you what element/organ is controlling the depleted one, taking energy away from it

A third way to balance the element:

After marking the five-element chart on the person's form.

Find the *main* element which is depleting *all* the other elements (there maybe two). Follow the arrows backward until you have an element with no mark in it. The element that is directly after the arrow with no mark, is the main element. Balance the organ in that element and all the other elements/organs should balance automatically.

CONTROLLING CYCLE

Wood consumes Earth

Earth dams Water

Water extinguishes Fire

Fire melts Metal

Metal cuts Wood

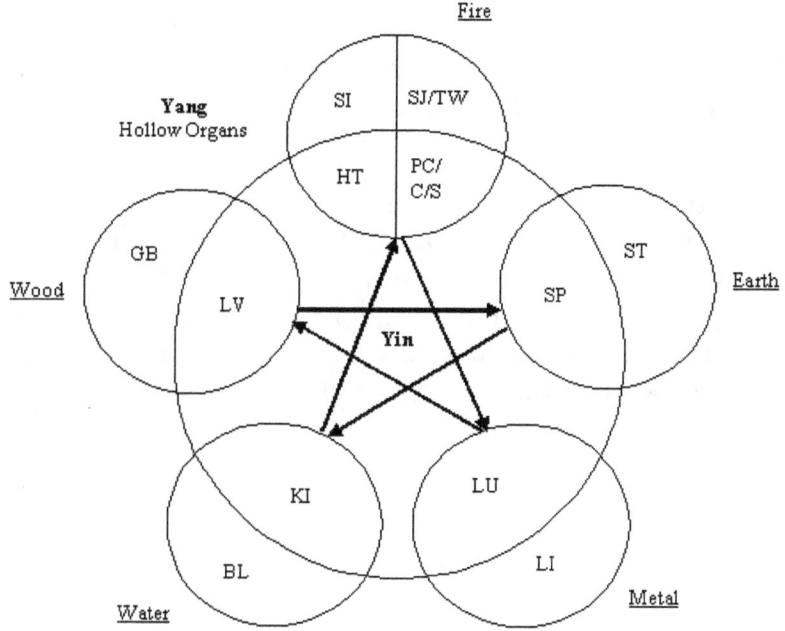

The five-element theory shows the relationship between the elements both nourishing and controlling. One element/organ can be deficient or in excess (out of balance) but if the dis-ease is chronic or been there for many years, in most cases, all of the elements will have been affected.

When doing a session and using the person's chart, you will test if someone has pain, dis-ease (emotional, physical, mental or spiritual) or wants to achieve a goal. You will muscle test each of the five elements, checking to see which are *off/yes* or not allowing the energy to flow freely using pulse reading, the person's arm or body pendulum technique.

This is where yang meridians (hollow organs) and yin meridians (always working organs) come in; you will now balance the body.

This is another way to balance the Meridians… Each of the five elements has characteristics, Nature and Human Body. Muscle test which of nature or human body balancing method you will be using.

The next few pages have the characteristic of the five elements. In these two sections (nature or human body) are other ways in which you may be able to balance the meridian/organ/element. For example, if the fire element is not in balance/off, you can muscle test to find out which of nature or human body characteristics is best to use to balance that meridian/organ/element.

FIRE
TRAITS AND CHARACTERISTICS

NATURE

Time of Day:	Midday
Season:	Summer
Natural Form:	Flame, Fire, Volcano, Sun
Process:	Growth
Climate:	Heat
Direction:	South
Color:	Red
Flavor:	Bitter
Smell:	Scorched

HUMAN BODY

Organ:	Heart and Small Intestine
Sense Organ:	Tongue
Sense:	Speech
Tissue:	Blood Vessels
Manifestation:	Face/Complexion
Fluid:	Perspiration
Sound:	Laughing
Emotion:	Joy, Happiness & Sorrow
Energy:	Expansive
Age:	Adolescence
Food	Garlic, Ginger, Fried onions, Onions, Mild spices, Oils, Corn, Nuts, Apricots, Seeds, Herbs, Moderately Coffee & Alcohol

EARTH
Traits and Characteristics

NATURE
Time of Day:	Afternoon
Season:	Late Summer & Last 10 days of each season
Natural Form:	Soil, Mountain, Rock
Process:	Ripening
Climate:	Humidity & Dampness
Direction:	Center
Color:	Yellow & Brown
Flavor:	Sweet
Smell:	Fragrant

HUMAN BODY
Organ:	Stomach and Spleen
Sense Organ:	Mouth
Sense:	Taste
Tissue:	Muscles, Flesh
Manifestation:	Lips
Fluid:	Saliva
Sound:	Singing
Emotion:	Compassion, Sympathy & Worry
Energy:	Downward
Age:	20's - 30's
Food:	Baked Potato, Baked Meals, Thick Soups, Bread

METAL
TRAITS AND CHARACTERISTICS

NATURE

Time of Day:	Evening
Season:	Autumn/Fall
Natural Form:	Minerals, Precious Metals, Crystals
Process:	Harvest
Climate:	Dryness (Cold)
Direction:	West
Color:	White
Flavor:	Spicy & Pungent
Smell:	Rotten

HUMAN BODY

DO NOT USE LI4 (HOKU) DURING PREGNANCY!

Organ:	Lungs and Large Intestine
Sense Organ:	Nose
Sense:	Smell
Tissue:	Skin
Manifestation:	Skin & Body Hair
Fluid:	Mucous
Sound:	Crying & Weeping
Emotion:	Grief & Melancholy
Energy:	Contracted
Age:	Middle Age (40's - 60s')
Foods:	Spicy, Rice, Mushrooms

WATER
TRAITS AND CHARACTERISTICS

NATURE

Time of Day:	Night
Season:	Winter
Natural Form:	Lake, Ocean, River, Rain, Snow, Cloud, Fog, Pond
Process:	Storage
Climate:	Cold (Dryness)
Direction:	North
Color:	Black & Blue
Flavor:	Salty
Smell:	Putrid

HUMAN BODY

Organ:	Kidney and Bladder
Sense Organ:	Ears
Sense:	Hearing
Tissue:	Bones
Manifestation:	Teeth, Bone Marrow, Bones, Head Hair
Fluid:	Urine
Sound:	Groaning
Emotion:	Fear
Energy:	Floating
Age:	Old Age (70's)
Food:	Salty, Watery Foods (Fish and Seafood), Drink Water

WOOD
TRAITS AND CHARACTERISTICS

NATURE

Time of Day:	Morning
Season:	Spring
Natural Form:	Trees, Grass, Plants, Flowers
Process:	Birth
Climate:	Wind
Direction:	East
Color:	Green
Flavor:	Sour
Smell:	Rancid

HUMAN BODY

Organ:	Liver & Gall Bladder
Sense Organ:	Eyes
Sense:	Sight
Tissue:	Ligaments & Tendons
Manifestation:	Nails
Fluid:	Tears
Sound:	Shouting
Emotion:	Anger
Energy:	Upward
Age:	Childhood
Food:	Meat, Green Vegetables, Sour Foods, Lemon & Lime

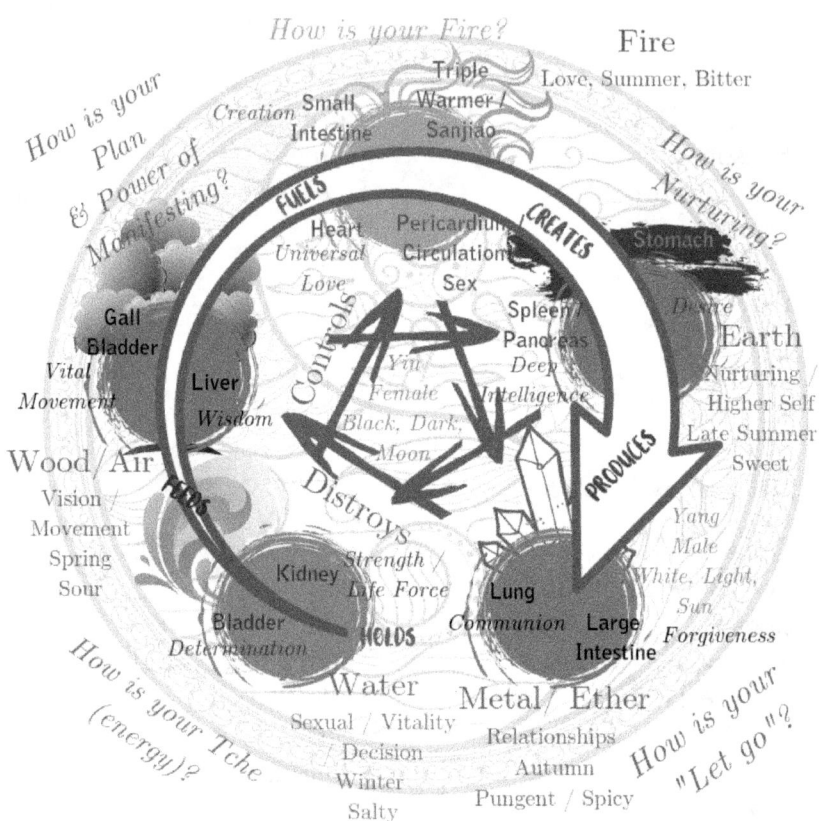

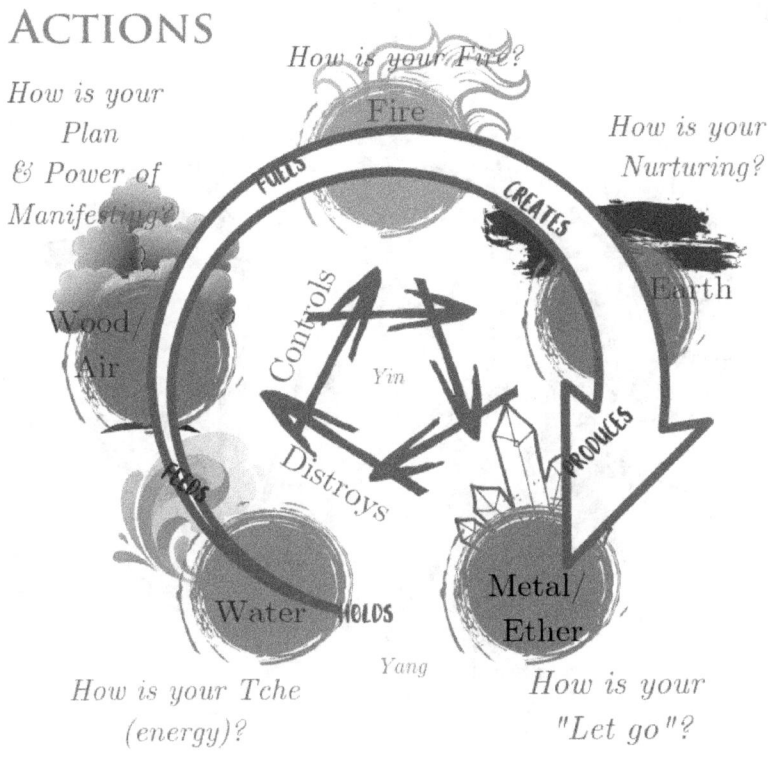

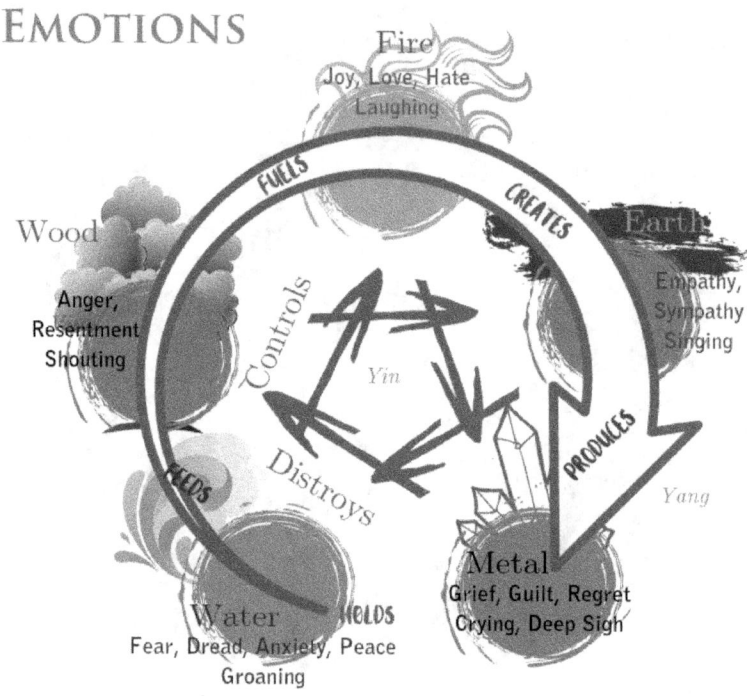

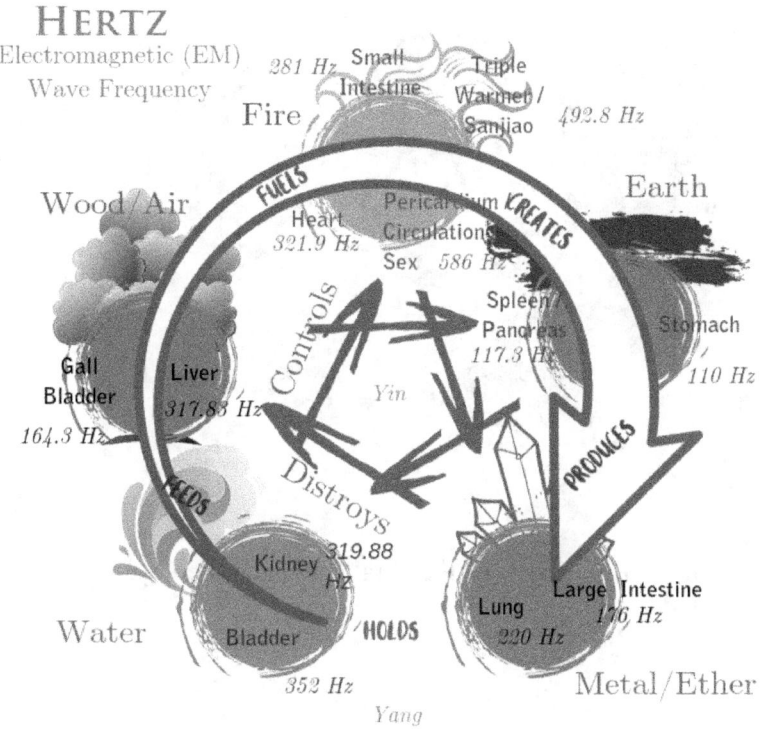

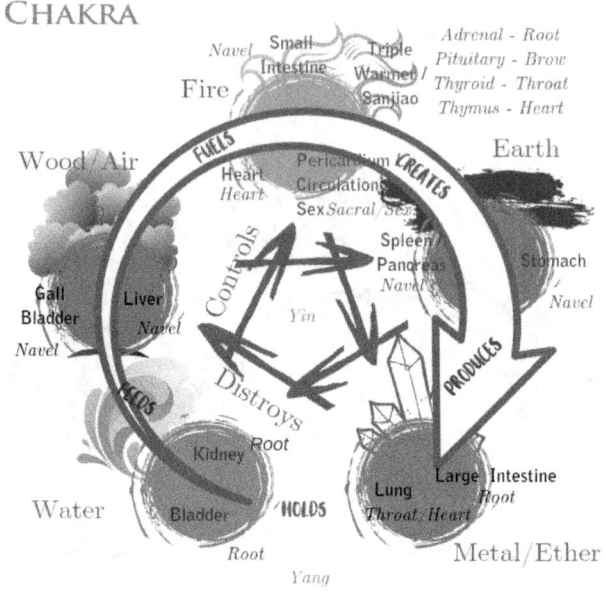

In Quantum Energy Medicine, the Vital Body and the Physical Body are connected through Chakras and Meridians.

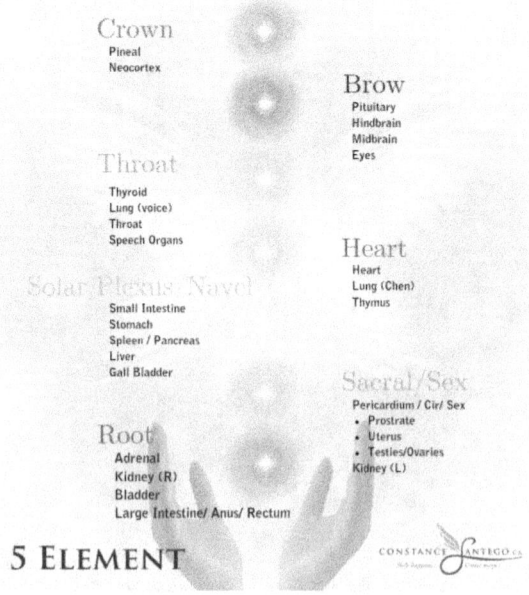

HOW TO PERFORM A SESSION

Step #1 Fill out a health form.
Step #2 Have the person choose an issue to work on; are they going to work on pain in their body or on a goal they would like to achieve?

The body senses 2-3million bits of information every second but only holds about 9 bits. Train your mind to retain what you want to create.

>*If a person chooses a goal. Write down the goal in the positive.

>>1- NO: e.g. I do not want to be fat or I am ugly (negative)

>>YES: I am my perfect weight, or I look good in pictures or I weigh_?_ lbs.   (positives)

>>2- NO: e.g. I want a nice car.

>The mind does not have enough specifics, so a nice car could be a Volkswagen when you really wanted a Jaguar.

>>YES: I own a beautiful red jaguar.

>>Or, I own a beautiful red jaguar that is in perfect condition.

>>Or, I own a beautiful red jaguar that is in perfect

condition and new.

> Or, I own outright a beautiful red jaguar that is in perfect condition and new.

Your mind will attract whatever you ask for.
Ever owned a car that was one color and then later you bought a different car that was a different color? What did you notice when driving the new car?... Notice how many cars are out there like yours and even the same color?

> Ever been in a very busy place waiting for someone? You were looking for him/her and there could be 100 people, but you easily spotted just the person for whom you were waiting.

*If pain is the issue; Have them tell you where the pain is and what the number is 1-10. 10 being a major pain. Mark this information down on the front or back of the body on the person's chart.

Step #3 Muscle test or pulse read which meridian is off. (Choice: you can muscle test the person's arm, have him/her body pendulum, use a surrogate person or pulse read).

Test all of the fourteen meridians, and circle *yes* or *no* on the chart.

Step #4 Transfer the answers to the Five Element Chart -onto the example of the chart we use.

Step #5 How did you balance the person? Muscle test which way is appropriate and then proceed to balance. To strengthen a yin or yang element/meridian/organ, you have many choices:

1) using the quick fix.

2) running meridian - 'zip-up' the meridian, which is not in balance, three times;

3) 'meridian walking the meridian which is not in balance;

4) using the source points;

5) strengthening or weakening the muscle (activate the muscle-origin /insertion);

6) making up your own (always muscle test to find out if it is appropriate);

7) going to a health professional (for example, a doctor or counselor).

Rule of balancing the five-element chart:

1) If Ren or Du is off-balance, balance first.

2) Check the Yin organs/meridians/elements - if two or more in a row are 'off', strengthen the first organ in the cycle and balance in clockwise order until all yin organs are strengthened.

3) Check the Yang organs/meridians/elements - if two or more in a row are 'off', strengthen the first organ in the cycle and balance in clockwise order until all yang organs are strengthened.

Step #6 Re-check goal or pain level. If it is pain, re-check the original spots on the body and write down the new number (one - ten), <u>circle</u> the new number.

Step #7 Check to see if the session is finished.

Step #8 Does the person need another session and, if yes, when?

Step #9 Homework: did you assign any homework to the person? (For example, you photocopied the quick fix in black and white and muscle tested the person to find out how often he does it himself.)

Step #10 If they are your client - Comments: anything you want to write down after the person leaves (for example, six children, loves his dog…)

*** If a person is not responding:

- **have him drink water.**

- **or, have him "zip-up" 3 times.**

- **or, have him use the washroom**

- **or, have him do the movement activity 5 times.**

OTHER QUESTIONS You Can Muscle Test:

1) Which system is best to work on first, second, etc. due to the health condition?

- Skeletal System — do any problems exist (some people see color, feel their own bodies reacting, just know what is wrong, or a voice tells them, make sure to write down whatever they tell you). The vertebral column, the human skull
- Muscular System — muscles
- Nervous System — Brain, hypothalamus, spinal cord, nerves
- Circulatory System — heart, arteries, veins,
- Urinary System — kidneys, bladder, ureter tube, urethra
- Reproductive System — women- uterus, ovaries, fallopian tubes, vagina men- prostrate, testicles, scrotum, seminal vesicles
- Digestive System — salivary glands, pharynx, esophagus, liver, gall bladder, duodenum, stomach, small intestine, pancreas, appendix, ascending colon, transverse colon, descending colon and rectum
- Endocrine System — pituitary gland, pineal, thyroid, parathyroid, thymus, adrenal, pancreas, ovaries, testes
- Immune & Lymphatic system — tonsils, sub-maxillary lymph nodes, axially lymph nodes, spleen, lymph vessels, lymph nodes, left thoracic duct, right

thoracic duct, inguinal lymph nodes
- Respiratory System — nose, trachea, bronchi, bronchioles, lung, diaphragm
- Sensory System- Eyes, Ears, Hair, Teeth, Skin,
    2. Is there a lesson for them to learn before they can cure this?
    3. At what age did this originate?
    4. Can you cure them?
    5. Is there something in your practice that can cure them?
    6. Can they cure themselves?
    7. Is there something in Kelowna that can cure them?
    8. Is there someone in Kelowna that can cure them?
    9. Is there something/someone in the world that can cure them?
    10. Is this caused by a product they use?
    11. Make-up, shampoo/conditioner, toothpaste, underarm deodorant, etc.
    12. Is it their medication that they are on?
    13. Is this caused by allergies?
    14. Is this caused by parasites?
    15. ETC.

2) If a person is really **Happy**: Muscle test what can make them even more happy.

Ideas:

Holiday, Seeing a friend or loved one, Spa Day, buy something, Anything that makes them happy!

3) If a person has **Muscle Pain:**

Do muscle-testing quick fix (1-10 pain level)

- If pain is <u>not</u> gone then do Energy Balancing or Reiki / Shiatsu / Swedish Massage
- If gone, muscle test a second, Happy or something else to work on

4) If a person is in **Emotional Pain**: Childhood, Sexual, etc.

Muscle test which session to do:

- Emotional Clearing Technique / Muscle testing
- Energy Balancing / Reiki
- Aromatherapy Blend
- Meditation
- Massage
- Go to another professional

5) If a person has a **Headache:**

Muscle test which session to do:

- Quick fix- muscle testing
- Aromatherapy essential oil blend
- Reflexology
- Table Shiatsu—acupressure points

6) If a person is in **Spiritual Pain**: Death in the family, Seeing, hearing, feeling or knowing things. Muscle test which session to do:

- Reiki
- Meditation
- Energy reading

7) If a person is in **Mental Pain**: Teacher, Accountant

Muscle test which session to do:

- Meditation
- Reiki
- Massage
- Reflexology

At the end of session muscle test date for the next session

EXTRA QUESTIONS:

8) Anything on -the right side of the body could be issues with males.

-the left side could be issues with females.

E.g. Left eye issues

Meaning – do not want to see anything; from Mom, themselves or women

Here are more ideas for literal questions for all four aspects of the body: Emotional, Mental, Physical and Spiritual

Start with asking this first: Emotional 'yes / no', Mental 'yes / no', Physical 'yes / no' or Spiritual 'yes / no' **(there may be more than one issue).**

EMOTIONAL:

Body

Mind — Musclologist

Soul — Social worker

Spirit — Psychiatrist

Person — Psychology

Place — Stress

Thing — Fears

Counseling — Phobias

Beliefs: Past__ Present__ Future__ Story Mode __

Emotional Clearing Technique

MENTAL:

Physical Brain- go to nervous system

Hemisphere:

    Left - analytical

    Right - creative

    Both – hemi-sync

Thoughts

    Conscious

    Subconscious

    Super conscious

Habit / Pattern

Reading

Writing

Comprehension

Speech

International Language

Communication:

    Audio, Visual, Feeler or Knower

Occupation

PHYSICAL:

Body Image

Climate

    Hot   Dry

    Cold   Wind

    Damp   Altitude

Pathogens__

  Fungi

  Virus

  Bacteria

  Parasite:

      Roundworms, Hookworm, Whipworm and Pinworm.

      Single Cell Parasites
          Protozoa, Cryptosporidium, Trichomonas, Vaginalis, Giardia

      Tapeworms
          Beef worm, Bladder worm, Pork Tapeworm, Broad fish Tapeworm, Dog Tapeworm, Dwarf Tapeworm, Rat Tapeworm.
      Flukes
          Liver, Lung, Blood flukes
      Spirochetes

Radiation

    Sun   Microwave

    Ultraviolet   Cell Phone

    Computer   Electrical

Contacts

    Detergent   Paint

    Soap   Solvents

    Deodorant   Chemicals

    Cosmetics   Materials

    Skin care

Breathing

Water

Scars

Cells

Chemical

    Vaccination

Medications _____

    Birth control

    Street Drugs _____

Injected

    Medications

    Supplements

Insulin

Bug bites

Senses: eyes, ears, smell, touch, taste

Allergies

Dairy	Vitamins
Grain	Minerals
Fruit	Chocolate
Vegetables	Coffee
Protein	Tea
Condiment	Nuts
Sugar	Caffeine
Alcohol	Molds
Supplement	

Additives

MSG coloring

Aspartame	Sulfur
Saccharine	Potassium
	Benzoate
Food	

Toxins

Pesticides	Phenol
Tobacco smoke	Redon
Perfume	Freon
Anesthetics	Methane
Fumes	Propane
Gasoline	Chlorine
Formaldehyde	Ammonia
	Carbon monoxide

Anatomy <u>Overview</u>

Cell

Circulatory	Nervous
Digestive	Reproductive
Endocrine	Respiratory
Immune	Skeletal
Lymphatic	Skin /Integument
Muscular	Urinary

Cell:

Nucleolus	Endoplasmic Reticulum
Nucleus	
Rough	Smooth

Endoplasmic Reticulum

Golgi Complex/Apparatus

Ribosomes

Secretory Vesicle

Lysosome

Vacuole

Mitochondria

Centrosome/Centrioles

Cytoskeleton

Cytoplasm

Cell Membrane

Cilia

Nuclear membrane

Circulatory:

Systemic / General Circulation
    Hepatic Portal
        Cardiac or Coronary
Pulmonary Circulation
Heart

    Blood

        Plasma
        Erythrocytes *(red blood corpuscles)*
            Oxyhemoglobin
            Carboxyhemoglobin
        Leucocytes *(white corpuscles)*
        Corpuscles Thrombocytes *(Platelets)*
        Thromboplastin
        Coagulation
    Subclavian arteries
    Axillary

Brachial
> PH level
>> Acid
>> Alkaline
> Blood type
> - A
> - B
> - AB
> - O
> - Rhesus positive or Rhesus negative

Beat

Blood Pressure

> Systolic pressure

> Rest-diastolic pressure.

Pericardium

Right and left Atriums

Right and left Ventricles

Ascending aorta

Aorta arch

Radial

Ulna

Palmer Arches.

Subclavian

Common Carotid

Facial

- Temporal
- Occipital
- Descending
- Thoracic Aorta
- Abdominal Aorta
- Iliac
- Femoral
- Popliteal
- Anterior Tibial
- Posterior Tibial
- Dorsalis Pedis
- Plantar Arches

Arteries
- Pulmonary artery
- Arterioles
- Capillaries

Veins
- Pulmonary vein
- Inferior vena cava
- Superior vena cava
- Venules
- Capillaries

Digestive System:

Taste

Appendix

Esophagus

Gallbladder

Liver

Pancreas

Teeth

Stomach

Small intestine

    Duodenum, Jejunum, Ileum

Large intestine

    Ileocecal valve, ascending colon, hepatic flexure, transverse colon, splenic flexure, descending colon, sigmoid flexure, sigmoid colon and rectum/anus

Endocrine System:

Hypothalamus

Adrenals

    Epinephrine (adrenaline), Norepinephrine, Endorphins, Cortisol, Aldosterone, DHEA

Pancreas

Insulin, Glucagon

Pineal

Melatonin

Ovaries or Testes

Testosterone, Estrogen, Progesterone

Pituitary

TSH, ACTH, FSH, LH, HGH, MSH, Endorphins, Prolactin, Growth hormone, Oxytocin, ADH

Thymus

Thymosin, thymine

Parathyroid

Thyroid

T3, T4, Calcitonin

Immune System:

Adenoids

Appendix

Spleen

Tonsils

Thymus

Monocytes

Megakaryocytes

Lymphocytes (B-Cells, T-cells)

Erythrocytes (red blood cells)

Antigens

    Immunoglobulins

    Complement proteins

    Cytokines

Lymphatic System:

Flow
Lymphocyte
    Bone marrow
    Thymus
Tonsils

Adenoids

Peyer's patches in the ileum

Spleen

    Red pulp

    White pulp

Appendix

Sub-maxillary

Lymph nodes

Axially lymph nodes

- Lymph vessels
- Lymph nodes
- Left thoracic duct
- Right thoracic duct
- Inguinal lymph nodes
- Popliteal fossa
- Cubical in the crutch of the elbow
- Sub clavicular glands,
- Submandibular glands
- Superficial cervical nodes
- Occipital nodes.

Muscular:

- Voluntary
- Involuntary
- Cardiac Muscle
- Endomysium
- Fascicles
- Perimysium
- Epimysium
- Filaments
- Muscle tone- agonist, antagonist

Tendon

Ligament

Waste- glucose, glycogen, fat lactic acid, carbon dioxide, heat and water

Head Muscles

Frontalis (or Epicranius)	Spinalis (or Spinatus)
Orbicularis Oculi	Latissimus Dorsi
Orbicularis Oris	Serratus Magnus
Masseter	Gluteus Maximus
Buccinator	Psoas
Sternocleido Mastoid	Pectoralis Major
Platysma	Abdominis Obliques
Trunk of Body	Abdominis Transversalis
Trapezius	Abdominis Rectus

Arms & Legs Muscles

Deltoid	Coraco Brachialis
Biceps Brachilias	Brachio Radialis
Triceps Brachialis	Pronator terres
Brachialis Anticus	Supinator

Flexor Carpi Radialis

Rectus Femoris

Vastus Lateralis (quadriceps)

Vastus Medialis (quadriceps)

Sartorius

Adductor Magnus

Longus and Brevis

Biceps Femoris (ham strings)

Semi-tendinosis

Semi-membranous

Gracilis

Gastrocnemius

Tibialis Anterior

Peroneus Longus

Flexor Digitorum

Tendon Achilles

Other_____

Nervous:

Blood / brain barrier

Efferent / Motor

Afferent / Sensory

Dendrites

Axon

Synapse

Neuron

Glial

Myelin sheath

Cellular sheath

Sciatic

Solar plexus

Brain –left, right

Central

Cortices-

Frontal

Parietal

Occipital

Temporal

Limbic-
Amygdala

Hippocampus

Fornix

Cingulate gyrus

Olfactory

Mammillary

Stria terminalis

Thalamus

Hypothalamus

Reptilian

Ventricles

Cerebellum

Basal Ganglia

Brain stem
(spinal column)

Midbrain

Pons

Medulla

Spinal cord

Peripheral

Somatic

Autonomic

sympathetic

parasympathetic

Reproductive:

Fallopian tubes

Ovaries

Ovum

Childbirth

Umbilical cord

Placenta

Water

Uterus

Fundus

Corpus

Cervix

Menstruation

Endometrium

Corpus luteum

Vagina

Vulva

Clitoris

labia

Breast

Penis

Prepuce

Corpus cavernosum

Prostate

Testes

Epididymis

Seminal vessel

Spermatic cord

Spermatozoon

Vas deferens

Cowper's Gland

Bulbourethral

Scrotum

Respiratory:

Smell / Olfactory

Lungs

Throat

Nose

Trachea

Bronchi

Bronchioles

Lung

Alveoli

Pharynx or Throat

Trachea or Windpipe

Bronchial tubes

Chest

Nose

Hair

Mucous membrane

Cilia

Macrophages

Larynx or Voice Box

Glottis

Epiglottis

Diaphragm

Phrenic nerves

Skeletal:

Yellow bone marrow

Red bone marrow

Osteoblasts

Osteoclasts

Long bone

Short bones

Flat bones

Irregular bones

Sesamoid bones

Joints

Sternum

Xiphoid process

Ribs

Ischium

Greater trochanter

Lesser trochanter

Innominate

Pubis

Girdle-

Sacrum

Coccyx

Ilium

Head-

Parietal, Temporal, Sphenoid, Nasal, orbit, Zygomatic, Frontal, Maxilla, Mandible, Occipital

Vertebrae-

Cervical, Thoracic, Lumber, Sacrum, Coccyx

Arm/Shoulder-

> Clavicle, Scapula, Acromion process, Humerus, Radius, Ulna, Carpal, Metacarpals, Phalanges

Legs-

> Femur, Patella, Tibia, Fibula, Tarsal, Metatarsal, Phalanges

Skin /Integument:

> Epidermis
>
> Dermis
>
> Subcutaneous layer
>
> Sebaceous glands
>
> Sudoriferous glands
>
> Apocrine sweat glands
>
> Exocrine sweat glands
>
> Hair Follicle
>
> Nails or onyx
>
> Motor nerve fibers
>
> Sensory nerve fibers
>
> Secretory nerve fibers

Urinary:

> Bladder
>
> Ureter
>
> Urethra
>
> Kidneys
>
> Cortex
>
> Middle Portion
>
> Pelvis

Senses
- Smell
- Touch
- Taste
- Common Sense
- Extra Sensory Perception
- Sight
- Hearing

SPIRITUAL:

Apport (paranormal) / Materialization

Astral Possession

Astral Projection / travel

Astral travel

Breath

Deep, Shallow

Channeling

Clairaudience

Claircognizance

Clairsentience

Clairvoyance

Dark Magic

Dreams

Prophetic

Dowsing

Extra Sensory Perception (ESP)

Impressions

Intuition

Karma

Medium

Paranormal Healing

Past live issue

Precognition / Premonition

Projection

Psychic Readings

Psychometry

Reincarnation

Remote Viewing

Scanner

Séance

Telepathy

Teleportation

Vibration

Human

Electrical

Chemical

Earth

Product

Mineral / Jewelry

Voodoo

Walk in

Psychic

Psychokinesis / Plant

Spirits / Apparitions

Hallucinations

Materializations

Human

Ghost / Poltergeist

Universe

Held

Hell

Human

Angel

Demon

Other _____

Elemental

    Fairies

    Fire (salamanders)

    Air (sylphs)

    Water (mermaids)

    Earth (gnomes & goblins)

Other _____

Heaven

Human

Guides

Guardian

Teacher

Worker

Protector

God (in any name)

Angels

Archangels

Gabriel

Michael

Uriel

Ascended Masters:

Ashtar

Count St. Germain

Dwal Kuhi

Jesus (Sananda)

Kuthumi

Mother Mary

Quan Yin

Serapis Bey

Other _____

Aura

Infected

Leaking

Muddy / Murky

Rip

Sharp

Soft

Tear

Other _____

The Etheric Body

The Emotional Body

The Mental Body

The Astral Body

The Etheric Template Body

The Celestial Body

The Ketheric Template Body

Memory Body, Soul Body, Integrative Body, Eternal Body and Universal Mind Body.

Complimentary color (Not true aura)

Color

    Red

    Orange

    Yellow

    Green

    Blue

    Indigo

    Violet

    Black

    White

    Grey

    Other _____

Spiritualism

    Belief

    Bible

Church

Cult

Item

Occult

Person

Prophets

Religion

Saints

Chakra

    Closed

    Semi open

    Open too much

Root / Base

Spleen / Sacral

Solar Plexus

Heart

Throat

Brow / Third Eye

Crown

Soul Star / Eight

Kundalini

Negative Energy

    Auto

    Building

    Room

    Place

    Thing

    Entity___

    Loved one

    Friend

    Enemy

    Negative / Positive

    Attachment

    Past life

    This life

    Job (was sent)

    Item (chair)

There are so many questions a person could ask...You will think of many more.

BIBLIOGRAPHY

Much of this information was created and copy written when I owned the Canadian Institute of Natural Health And Healing Accredited College

John Thie (1979) Touch for Health: A Practical Guide to Natural Health Using Acupressure Touch and Massage (Spiral-bound)

Andrew Biel (4th Edition 2010) Trail Guide to the Body: How to Locate Muscles, Bones and More. Books of Discovery

Robert Frost (2002) Applied Kinesiology – A Training Manual and Reference Book of Basic Principles and Practices. North Atlantic Books

F.M. Houston, DC (1974) The Healing Benefits of Acupressure. Keats

Angela Hicks (1996) Thorson's Principles of Chinese Medicine. Thorson

Susan L. Levy, DC and Carol Lehr, MA (1996) Your Body Can Talk, How to Use Simple Muscle Testing To Learn What Your Body Knows And Needs. HOHM Press

Anodea Judith (1996) Eastern Body Western Mind, Psychology And Chakra System As A Path To The Self. Celestial Arts

Gerry Thompson (1994) The Shiatsu Manual, Step-by-step techniques for a full body treatment. Sterling Publishing Co

Body Talk www.thebodytalkclinic.com

Courses: Touch for Health, Taught By Evelyn Mulders
Body Talk, Taught by Kristy Kenny
Aromatic Kinesiology, Taught by Robbi Zeck ND

Chart: Acupuncture Points (1996-2010) Permacharts.com

P.S.S. There are scientific machines out there that will beep when you pass over a tsubo on a meridian point in your body.

http://www.jinshindo.org/meridians

MESSAGE FROM THE AUTHOR

Muscle Testing is probably the most brilliant form of self-empowerment that any one person could develop and use.

Try out the techniques I have listed in this manual and master at least one that you can trust for accuracy. Use Muscle Testing to make any of your easy and hard decisions.

JUST REMEMBER it is the question that you ask that is more important than the answer that you receive. The more literal the question the higher accuracy of the answer

Test this on you, your family, friends, career, education, entertainment. . . anything!

Have fun!!!

Constance

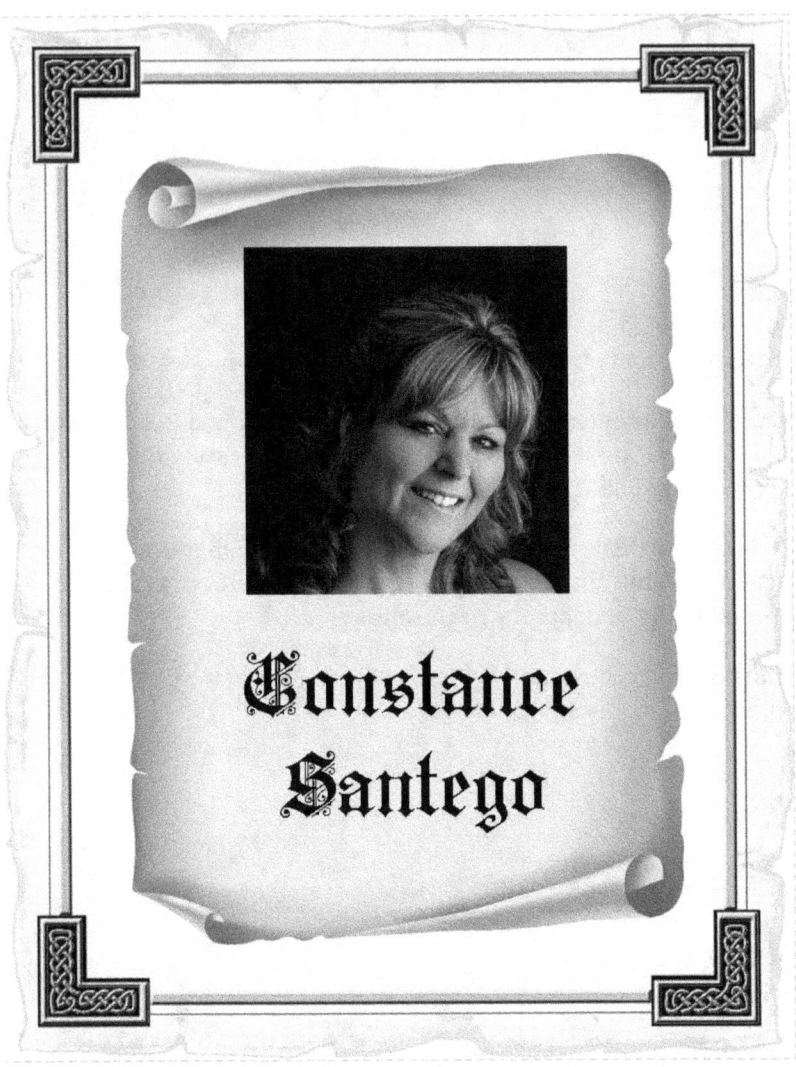

Muscle Testing
is what saved my body from pain, my mind from stress and my soul from insanity. I do not know what physical, emotional, mental or spiritual state I would be in if it was not for learning this modality…the magic of muscle testing!!!

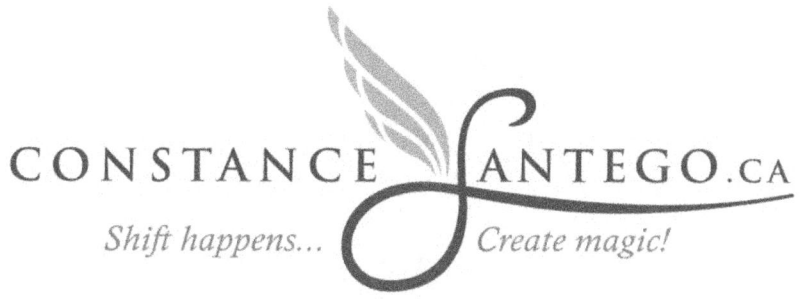

Constance Santego is a Master Educator, Author, and Holistic Spiritual Coach. She is known for bridging the body, mind, and soul consciousness to create your dreams into reality.

Constance's background is in business, owning her first company at the age of twenty-seven until her back went out and she had to sell. Learning how to heal herself holistically, she gained many, many certificates and diplomas in spirituality and natural healing.

Connie believes that the practice of the healing arts, open a gateway of quantum energy, and that is where the real magic takes place. If a study is teachable to others anywhere in the world, then science is involved and becomes fact.

The nine spiritual gifts from the Bible has been taught for over two thousand years. The Secrets of a Healer Series is based on the 'Spiritual Gift of Healing.'

Constance continually strives to advance her knowledge and is currently in the process of attaining her Ph.D. and DOCTORATE in Natural and Integrative Medicine.

www.ingramcontent.com/pod-product-compliance
Lightning Source LLC
Chambersburg PA
CBHW050554300426
44112CB00013B/1905